Ana Rita Barcessat
Luciana Corrêa

Oncological photodynamic therapy

Ana Rita Barcessat
Luciana Corrêa

Oncological photodynamic therapy

Considerations in cell death and proliferation

ScienciaScripts

Imprint

Cover image: www.ingimage.com

This book is a translation from the original published under ISBN 978-3-330-76884-0.

Publisher:
Sciencia Scripts
is a trademark of
Dodo Books Indian Ocean Ltd. and OmniScriptum S.R.L publishing group

120 High Road, East Finchley, London, N2 9ED, United Kingdom
Str. Armeneasca 28/1, office 1, Chisinau MD-2012, Republic of Moldova, Europe
Managing Directors: Ieva Konstantinova, Victoria Ursu
info@omniscriptum.com

Printed at: see last page
ISBN: 978-620-8-60061-7

SUMMARY

Chapter 1 - Introduction to photodynamic therapy - PDT

1.1 Concepts of Photodynamic Therapy

Alternative therapies, also known as complementary and integrative therapies, such as cryotherapy, sonodynamic therapy, phytotherapy and photodynamic therapy have been studied for the treatment of various tumors[1]. *Photodynamic* therapy (PDT), which has been used in oncology since 1903 for basal cell carcinomas, is based on a photochemical reaction that generates reactive oxygen species, invalidating cells in the vicinity of the reaction, with no obvious genotoxic effects[2,3]. The mechanism is based on a triad involving a photosensitizing substance, light and tissue oxygen. Through death cascades that are still unclear, it is capable of rendering cells with significant metabolic alterations unviable. The therapy can also be used for antimicrobial purposes, consisting of using the properties to promote the death of microorganisms through the same oxidative effect[1-3].

Studies have focused on the effectiveness of the photodynamic effect, based on the chemical improvement of photosensitizers, their combinations with light at wavelengths suitable for penetration into biological tissues and compatible with the absorption spectrum of the photosensitizer, as well as efficient lighting protocols, in addition to studies of cell death mechanisms derived from PDT. [4]

The acute inflammatory process and the non-specific innate tumor immunity triggered by PDT have already been explained, but still require further clarification, for example in relation to the participation of mast cells. Tumor vascular reactions seem to be another crucial point in the biological mechanism of PDT due to the irreversible photoxidative damage to the microcirculation, causing hypoxia and a reduction in tumor volume, due to the affinity of certain photosensitizers to endotheliocytes.[5]

Factors related to the technique, the tumor and the host will interfere directly in the effectiveness of the photodynamic effect, so that the best of each aspect must be worked out for the greatest clinical benefit.

The prospects for PDT cancer therapy were established in the second decade of the 21st century, in the study and clinical development of photoconjugates and nanotechnology in photosensitizers.[5]

1.2 **Historical Principle** :

Studies using light to prevent and treat diseases are intertwined with the very history of civilizations: in ancient Egypt and India, over four thousand years ago, there were already indications of the treatment of vitiligo through the association of the ingestion of plants containing photoactive substances such as psoralens, furocoumarins and benzofurans (*Psoralea corylifolia*) associated with sun exposure. Over the years, ultraviolet light has been used to treat tuberculosis and *Lupus vulgari*, and Niels Finsen (Nobel Prize in Medicine, 1903) used red light to prevent variola and treat cutaneous tuberculosis, however, it was at the end of the 19th century in Germany, in a study of the toxicity of red acridine in parameciums, that the scientist Oscal Raab, a pupil of Herman Von Tappenier, observed that this dye in combination with light caused the death of the protozoa. At the same time as the French neurologist Prime used eosin to treat epilepsy, it caused dermatitis in areas exposed to the sun, leading to studies associating eosin with white light to treat skin tumors, Tappenier, in partnership with the German scientist Jodlbauer, later demonstrated the need for oxygen in these reactions, and at that time, 1904, the term *photodynamic* reaction *(photodynamische erscheinung)* was used for the first time [2)].

In 1913, Friederich Meyer-Betz injected porphyrin (later called hematoporphyrin), diluted in sodium hydroxide and saline solution, which showed strong and long-lasting photosensitivity after exposure to sunlight, becoming the initial milestone in human treatment with porphyrin[3].

In the 1920s, Policard studied porphyrins in tissues, observing their high concentrations via fluorescence in malignant tumors[4]. The fifties and sixties of the 20th century mark the history of the first generation of photosensitizers, basically porphyrins, for PDT with the studies of Schwartz, who found that Meyer-Betz had not injected pure porphyrin as he thought, because this compound is eliminated by the body very easily, but an oligomeric mixture which he called HpD, i.e. derivatives of hematoporphyrins[3,4].

In 1960, Lipson, under the guidance of Schwartz, verified through fluorescence the preferential accumulation of these derivatives in rodent tumor xenotransplants, and also observed regression of the lesion after irradiation, These trials would later lead him to publish a case report of a successful treatment of breast cancer, using HpD with selective irradiation of the tumor by visible light, which would characterize one of the first photodiagnostic trials, as well as the beginning of photodynamic therapy in the clinical treatment of cancer. Dougherty in 1975, using HpD and red light, stopped the growth of breast cancer in mice and also later described PDT with an argon laser [5].

The following year it was postulated, through the studies of Weishaupt and collaborators, that the singlet oxygen molecule, generated from the energetic transfer of a given agent in an excited state (triplet) to tissue oxygen, was responsible for the cytotoxicity and invalidation of tumor cells, at the same time that the first tests on patients using HpD occurred in bladder cancer with JF Kelly [(6).]

About twenty years passed before the first drug derived from hematoporphyrin was approved by the American FDA (Food and Drug Administration - USA) for commercial use in 1998, Photofrin® (porfimero sodium), which was developed from improvements based on Dougherty's experiments, by a Canadian company, for systemic PDT use in cancer and then Levulan® Kerastick (5-aminolevulinic acid - ALA) for the treatment of dermatological lesions. Another porphyrin derivative, a benzoporphyrin under the trade name Visudyne (veteporfin), was released for PDT in the treatment of macular degeneration of the retina due to the effect of the therapy on blood vessels in 2000 and temoporfin, under the trade name Foscan ®, was released in 2001 for head and neck cancer therapy [5-6]. The 21st century has been marked by improvements in the properties of photosensitizers and light sources in association with optical fibers, allowing us to work in depth on the development of the third generation of photosensitizers derived from porphyrins, as well as non-porphyrinic photosensitizers, conjugated to antibodies (photoimmunoconjugates) and liposomal nanoparticles, investing in the system for delivering the Fs to the tissue and increasing its selectivity [7]. Figure 1 schematically illustrates the timeline of PDT over the centuries.

Figure 1 - Photodynamic therapy over time

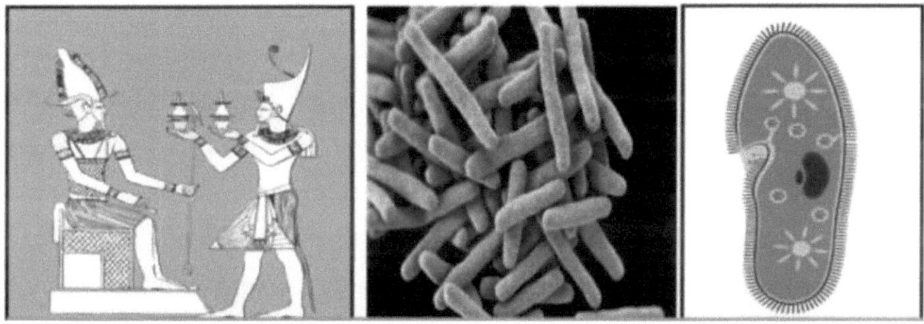

Plants and photoactive substances in ancient Egypt | go ; Light on bacteria and protozoa, 19th century Europe.

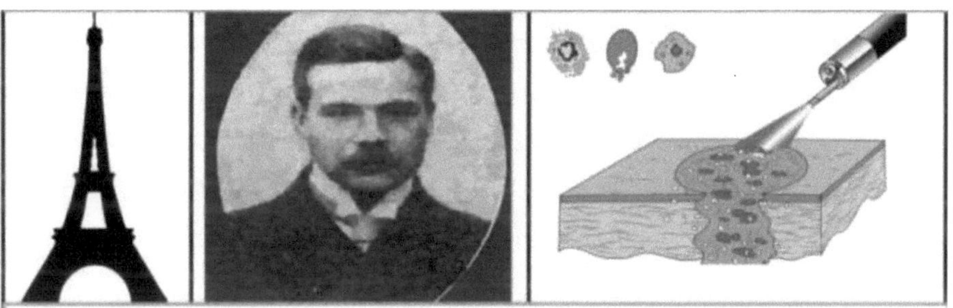

20th century Europe: eosin and dermatitis in sun-exposed areas Friederich Meyer - Betz photosensitivity after self-injection of hematoporphyrin; fluorescence in malignant tumors

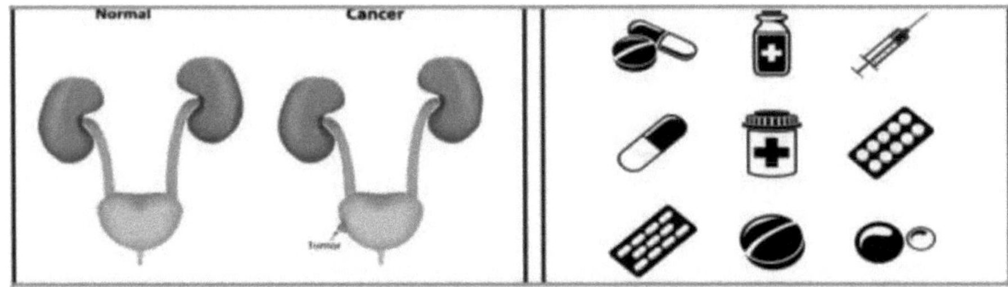

After the 1950s: America and Europe: application to human tumors and development of commercial photosensitizers

Source : **personal archive**[3]

1.3 General principles

The principle of the technique is based on the fact that the interaction of light with a compound of low toxicity in the dark (photosensitizer - Fs) and endogenous oxygen ($^{3}o_{2}$) results in reactive oxygen species (ROS), which, when in excess and above the anti-oxidation limit, are capable of invalidating cells or microorganisms [5]. Fs accumulates selectively in tumor areas (with greater metabolic activity), which causes the death of altered cells, with little or no damage to normal cells. It is characterized as a physical-chemical method for the local treatment of cancer or potentially malignant lesions, as well as for microbial reduction, which has been used in patients with tumours of small size and/or for whom conventional oncological therapy is proving to be ineffective or not indicated, or to reduce the size of the lesion, making subsequent surgery possible [6]. The indication for PDT will depend directly on the type of photosensitizer used and its properties; the light source and its combination with the Fs will determine the photodynamic effect when combined with tissue oxygen [5].

1 Illustration Sandro Souza Limeira da Silveira , comic book artist

Chapter 2 - Mechanisms

2.1 - Mechanism of Photodynamic Therapy - PDT

PDT consists of the association of an Fs, colloquially called a dye, with resonant electromagnetic energy and oxygen, which generates a photodynamic effect, i.e. the Fs absorbs photons from the light source and its electrons then pass into an excited (higher energy) but unstable state, called the singlet state (S^n) [8]. Figure 2 shows a schematic representation of this mechanism.

Figure 2 - Triad of Photodynamic Therapy - PDT

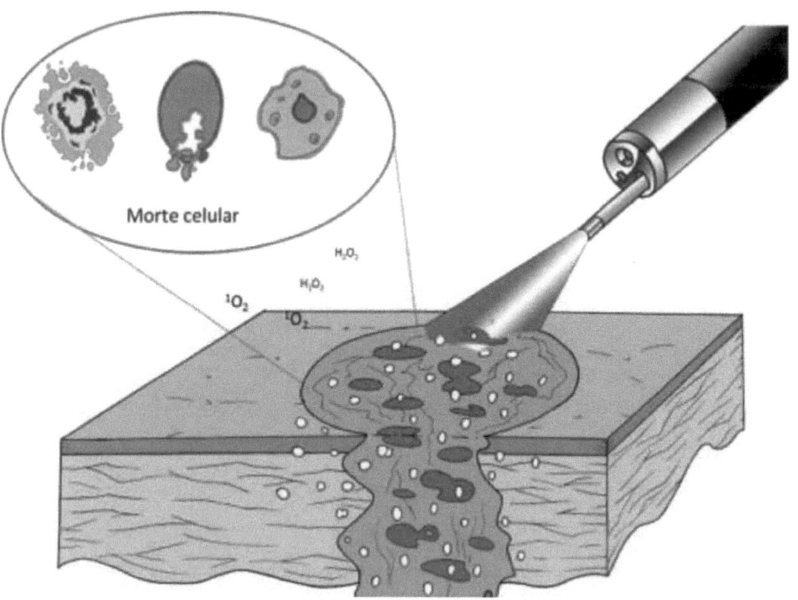

Figure 2 - PDT triad represented by the photosensitizing substance, light and tissue oxygen. This combination generates reactive oxygen species ($^1O_2$), cytotoxic molecules capable of invalidating cells by activating various mechanisms. **Source: personal archive**, illustration by Sandro Souza.

The excited Fs molecule will either lose energy and return to the ground state (S^0) emitting fluorescence, or, by spin inversion, it will reach a lower energy state called the "triplet" (T^1), which has a longer lifetime (in the order of µs-ms)[9]. At this stage, the photosensitizer molecule can: a) again undergo electronic decay and return to the fundamental level (S^0); b) undergo reduction and oxidation reactions with its environment through the transfer of electrons to components of the system, generating short-lived radical ions, called reactive oxygen species (ROS), which tend to react with oxygen in the fundamental state ($^3O_2$), resulting in oxidized products (a phenomenon known as type I reaction); or c) transfer their excitation energy to molecular oxygen ($^3O_2$), which leads to the formation of singlet oxygen ($^1O_2$), an unstable, highly reactive and cytotoxic molecule with a very short half-life (less than 40 ns) and an action radius of approximately 20 nm (a phenomenon known as type II reaction)[(8-10)] (Figure 3).

Figure 3 - Type I and type II reactions

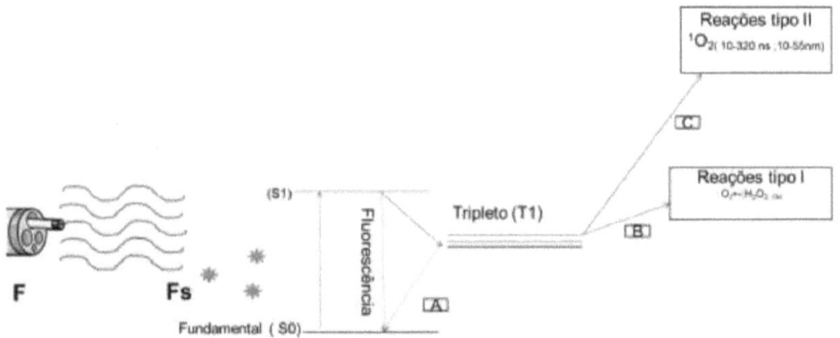

Figure 3 - Type I and type II reactions. The photosensitizer (Fs), activated by a light source (F) of a compatible wavelength, leaves the ground state (S0) and enters the excited state (S1). The excited molecule will either lose energy and return to the ground state (S0), emitting fluorescence, or descend to the triplet state (T1), which can (a) decay to S0, (b) generate reactive oxygen species (ROS) forming oxidized products when they react with molecular oxygen ($^3O_2$) or (c) directly transfer energy to $^3O_2$ forming singlet oxygen ($^1O_2$). Jablonski diagram adapted. **Source : created by the authors with adaptation.**[7]

One of the ROS that arise from type I reactions is the superoxide anion (O_2^-), which can be enzymatically converted into hydrogen peroxide (H_2O_2) and oxygen (O_2), in a reaction catalyzed by the enzyme superoxide dismutase (SOD)[11-12]. The superoxide anion and other EROS, together with singlet oxygen, function as oxidizing molecules that react readily with molecules in the biological system, modifying, by oxidative reactions, residues of amino acids and unsaturated lipids, or even damaging DNA when they reach the cell nucleus 9, [13-1]5.

Depending on the subcellular location of the EROS, the oxidative effects are transformed into adaptive responses or cell death 16. Cell damage occurs directly through the accumulation of Fs in vital intracellular targets such as the plasma membrane, mitochondrial membranes, endoplasmic reticulum cisternae, Golgi complex and lysosomes. There is no consensus that Fs accumulates in the cell nucleus, which indicates that PDT does little damage to nuclear DNA 14,1[7].There is evidence that Fs accumulation in mitochondrial membranes and the endoplasmic reticulum induces apoptosis processes, while this cascade is blocked when this accumulation occurs in the membrane or lysosomes, inducing cell necrosis. There are also indications that autophagy is activated in the cell as a form of defense against the spread of the deleterious effects of EROS to the organelles after irradiation[14,16,18].

The photodynamic effect is always dependent on the triad Fs, resonant electromagnetic energy and tissue oxygen, so that these elements generate minimal alterations to the tissues when used in isolation[4] (Figure 2).

Fs accumulates selectively in areas of greater metabolic activity, which causes the destruction of altered cells with little damage to normal cells [19].As most Fs are located in membranes, lipids are the main targets of EROS. Because of this preference for lipids, most Fs have a preference for mitochondrial membranes, which are abundantly found in tumor cells and also in the microvascular framework [20].

Direct tumor cell damage is not the only way in which PDT manifests its effects, damage to the tumor vascular network seems to be of great relevance to cell death by hypoxia, as well as significant changes in tumor immunity patterns 21. Thus, in summary, the basic triad of the photodynamic reaction is formed: the photosensitizer, oxygen and light. This combination generates a high local cytotoxic effect when it exceeds cellular antioxidant limits, whether in a tumor cell, a bacterial cell or a cell infected with a virus, with direct effects on macromolecules, activating cascades of different types of cell death.

2.2 **Types of Photodynamic Therapy: Oncological PDT and Antimicrobial PDT**

Oncological and antimicrobial PDT use the same principle of oxidative stress, PDT with the purpose of killing microorganisms has resurfaced due to the great microbial resistance to drugs that has developed in recent decades, some differences between Fs for the photodynamic effect on tumor cells and microorganisms are pointed out in table 1 below:

Table 1- Comparison between the different applications of PDT

Oncology PDT	**Antimicrobial PDT**
lipophilic Fs	Hydrophilic
Fs with low overall load	Cationic
High absorption bands (infrared / red) for high tissue penetration	No need to penetrate, superficial infections

Source : Adapted [22]

The more charges, i.e. the more cationic, the more effective the Fs are at targeting gram-negative bacteria [7,8,22].

The use of PDT will trigger death mechanisms in both cells and microorganisms. EROS in contact with intracellular targets, even with the lipids in viral capsids, even with the envelope of fungi and parasites, can trigger the rupture of their membranes, with the consequent release of intracellular material and necrosis, rendering the cell in question unviable. The same reasoning applies to the tumor vascular network and tumor cells, however, it will also depend on the selectivity of the photosensitizer. Figure 4 is a hypothetical representation of EROS on various cellular targets.

Figure 4 - Reactive Oxygen Species and cellular targets

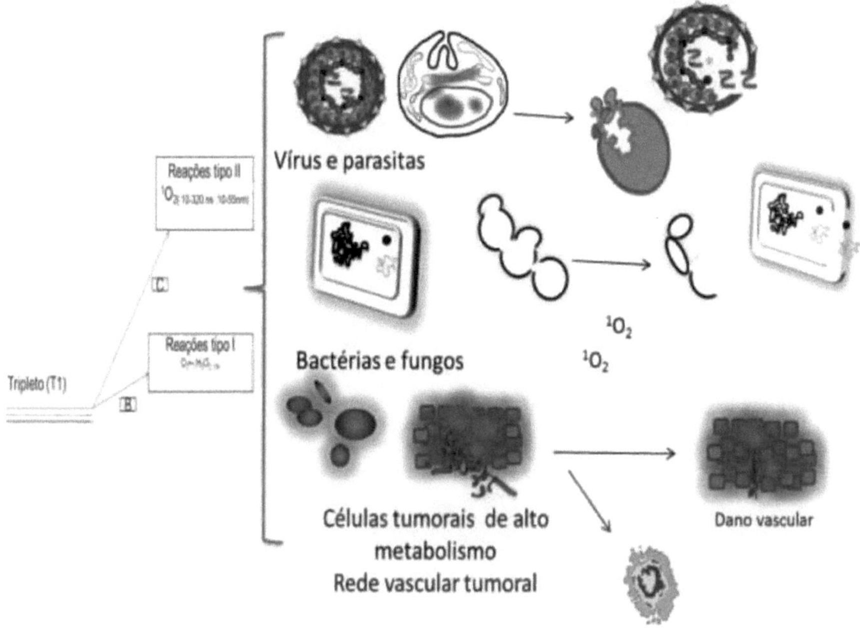

Figure 4 - Representative diagram of the reactive oxygen species (ROS) resulting from type I and II photodynamic reactions on the cells, tissues and microorganisms in which they act.

Source : created by the authors with adaptation [20-22]

CHAPTER 3 - Photosensitizers for use in photodynamic therapy

3.1 General Characteristics of Fs :

The photosensitizer is the photosensitive substance that, in contact with the photons from the light source, reaches a state of higher energy and transfers it to tissue oxygen, generating type I and type II reactions (figures 3 and 4). The challenge in oncological PDT is to have a photosensitizer with low toxicity to healthy tissues and high selectivity for tumor cells, thus establishing a drug suitable for each tumor type[9] ,12, [1]3, [(15)].

The appropriate amount of the drug to be used and the pre-irradiation time are important data to consider, in addition to factors relating to the light source, such as the type of source, the energy density, for example, which should be individualized for each application.22

A striking feature of FS for oncological use is their selectivity for tumor cells compared to non-tumor cells, even when applied systemically 21.

High lipophilicity for quick and easy penetration of biological barriers and high efficiency in the production of reactive oxygen species are also desirable conditions, especially for applications in oncology [23].

FS must be stable when stored, they must be active in the absence of light and necessarily harmless to normal tissues, they must have a short half-life and rapid elimination from tissues and also have high solubility in water, in injection vehicles and solutions and in blood constituents, facilitating their penetration and diffusion for systemic applications [21, 24].

The pre-irradiation time should be short between administration and maximum cellular accumulation in the region to be treated 23, which in turn will depend on the lipophilic properties of the Fs , however this idea has not always been consensual , for systemic applications, it used to be recommended to use a long irradiation interval in order to eliminate the Fs from healthy cells, but the most current argument is based on the reasoning that with a shorter interval it is possible to promote vascular damage by irradiating the endotheliocytes while there is still Fs in these cells [22].

The more polar the compound, the slower its penetration into cells, as it tends to follow adsorptive or endocytosis processes, requiring a longer irradiation interval [20,22].In this way, subcellular localization ends up being more important than the quantity of the photosensitizer in the photodynamic response, since the effect is local, for example, Fs with an affinity for plasma and mitochondrial membranes, such as porphyrins, will be more effective in inducing cell death than those which remain dispersed in the cytosol, such as phenothiazines [25 26].

3.2 The Paramètres of the light source :

It is known that it is necessary to use light with a resonant frequency with the optical absorption level of the Fs. Ribeiro *et al* [27] established the probability of energy transfer from the Fs to the tissue oxygen at a resonant frequency ω0, see figure 5.

Figure 5- Probability of energy transfer from FS to tissue oxygen

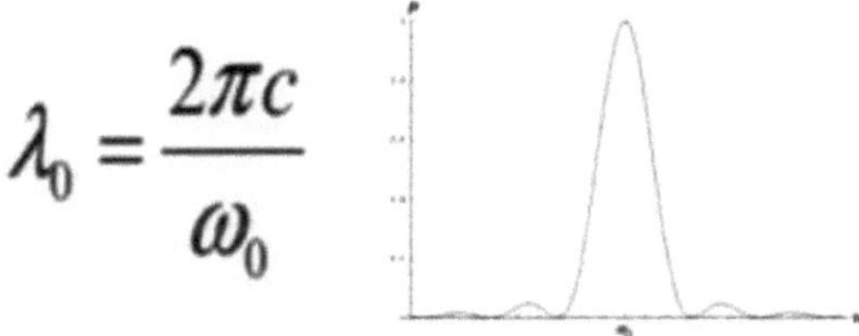

$$\lambda_0 = \frac{2\pi c}{\omega_0}$$

Figure 5 - c is the speed of light, at which the probability of energy transfer from Fs to triplet oxygen is close to 1, dropping considerably as you move away from this resonant frequency.

Source : Ribeiro *et al*, 2005, p.5 [27]

There is therefore a suitable wavelength to activate the photodynamic process and generate EROS, which should be a light with the appropriate power density and energy, preferably collimated and with a LONG wavelength, according to the formula (Figure 5). These characteristics favor laser sources, which are not, however, the only ones possible in PDT [27].

The fractionation of the energy delivered to the tissue is still a factor to be studied, so that low, fractionated doses could allow the renewal of oxygen levels to potentiate the photodynamic effect, since high power densities excite a large part of the Fs quickly in a short period of time [21]. Another issue to consider, especially in topical applications, is the ability of the light to penetrate the skin. There is no rigorous mathematical model of transcutaneous light penetration, precisely because of the irregularity and anatomical variability of this organ [24,28].

Depending on its precise chemical structure, an effective photosensitizer can be synthesized with an absorbance between 600 and 800 nm [22]. Thus, one of the characteristics of an ideal photosensitizer for "*in vivo*" application *is that it* has a maximum absorption of light *in* the red region of the visible light spectrum (650 to 780 nm). This characteristic is desirable because it makes it possible to avoid light absorption by endogenous pigments such as hemoglobin, which is strongly absorbed between 400 and 600 nm. Wavelengths in the 400 nm range do not penetrate sufficiently into the tissues to generate the photodynamic effect and those above 1000 nm produce molecular vibration leading to photothermal effects, not providing enough energy to raise the oxygen to its singlet state [20-22]. Figure 6 schematically represents the penetration of some wavelengths into the skin.

Figure 6 - Hypothetical schematic representation of the penetration of some light wave frequencies into tissues.

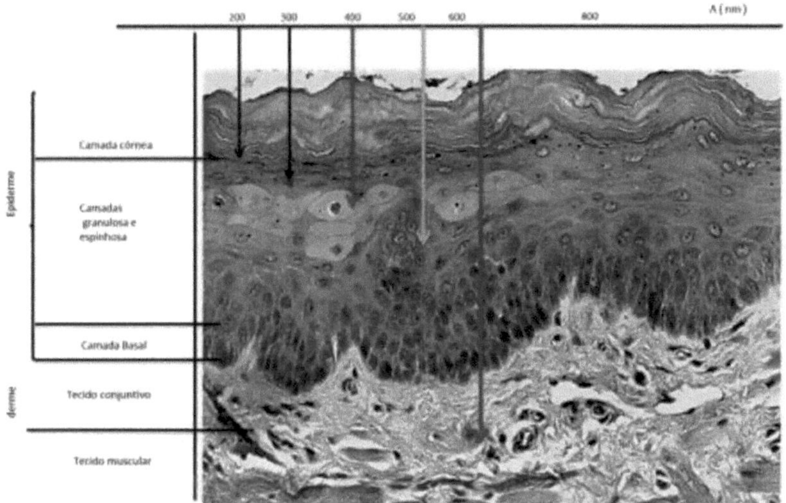

Figure 6 - Blue light (in the 400 nm range) and ultra violet light (around 200400 nm) penetrate little into tissues, while red and infrared light reach deeper layers.

Source : Created by the authors with adaptation [28]

It can then be seen that the transcutaneous penetration of light increases in proportion to the wavelength, and compounds such as chlorines, bacteriochlorines and phthalocyanines with strong absorbance in the red region of the light spectrum tend to be more effective photosensitizers, although this is not the only factor to consider. [21,22] On the other hand, it is important to note that the energy of singlet oxygen is approximately 94 $kJ.mol^{-1}$, which corresponds to the energy of 1270 nm. However, wavelengths longer than 800 nm are rarely used in PDT due to the high degree of scattering in tissues and the absence of a photosensitizer that absorbs in this region of the spectrum [29].

Even with the same Fs, no light source is ideal for all PDT applications, so the choice of source should be based on the absorption of the Fs (action spectrum and fluorescence) and the disease (location and size of lesions, access and tissue characteristics).[21]

3.3 Types of Photosensitizers and oncological use in PDT :

Table 2 - Some photosensitizers in PDT

Tetrapyrroles		
Porphyrins (and ALA)	Chlorines/bacteriochlorines	Phthalocyanines
HpD	Temoporfin or Foscan	chlorinated aluminium sulphonated phthalocyanines (CASPs)
Photofrin	benzoporphyrin derivative (Verteporfin	Zinc phthalocyanine
	Radachlorin (Bremachlorin)	PC4- phthalocyanines siliconized
	Chlorine(e6) - photodithazine; Monoaspartyl derivative (laserphyrin, sodium taloporphin or LS11)	RLP068 Cationic phthalocyanines
	Bacteriochlorins Palladium-bacteriofeoforbide bacteriophaeophorbide - TOOKAD LUZ11[4]	
Synthetic dyes		
Phenothiazines	Squaraine, Xanthenes, triphenylmethanes Rose	boron-dipyrromethene(BODIPY)

[4] Photodynamic Therapy With LUZ11 in Advanced Head and Neck Cancer, Clinical Trials.Gov NCT02070432

	Bengal (xanthene)	
Methylene blue	Squarine	
Toluidine blue	Malachite Green (triphenylmethane)	
PP904		
EtNBS (benzophenothiazinic)		
Natural products		
Perylenelequinone pigments	Riboflavin (vitamin B12)	Curcumin (saffron)
Hypericin		
Hypocrelin A and B		
Metals and others		
Furelenes	Titanium dioxide (nanoparticulate)	

Source : Created by the authors with adaptation [21,22, 30-35]

Photosensitizers can be classified according to their chemical structure as porphyrinic (with a tetrapyrrolic nucleus) and non-porphyrinic. Porphyrins and their derivatives are further categorized into first, second and third generations, as shown in Table 3. Non-porphyrinic photosensitizers, on the other hand, include texafirins, porphyrins, phthalocyanines and naphthalocyanines [22, 23, 24, 30-35]

Table 3: Oncological Use of Photosensitizers for Photodynamic Therapy

Generation	**Photosensitizer**	**Activation length**	**Employment**
First generation	Hematoporphyrin (Hp) Hematoporphyrin derivatives (HpD) and	630 nm	solid tumors: lung, stomach, esophagus, cervix, skin [36,38,39]

	Photofrin		
Monday	Palladium-	763 nm	lung cancer [37]
Generation	bacteriofeoforbide (TOOKAD)		
	meso-tetrakis-hydroxyphenylchlorine - m- THPC (Foscan® Temoporfin®) Photoditazine (PDZ)-mono-L-aspartyl chlorine	652 nm	Head and neck squamous cell carcinoma [38].
	BPD- MA - ring benzoporphyrin A monoacid derivative (Verteporfin, Visudyne ®)	690 nm	macular degeneration, choroidal hemangioma[39] sentinel lymph node (experimental) [40]
	5-aminolevulinic acid - ALA (Levulan ®, Alacare, Amulux)	635 nm	Head and neck squamous cell carcinoma [36' 38,41]
	ALA methyl ester (Metvix®) Benzyl ester of ALA (Benzvix)	635 nm	Skin, bladder, esophagus Adenocarcinomas gastrointestinal tract [42,43]
	Talaporfin sodium, NPe6, mono-L-	664 nm	Solid organ tumors

	aspartylchlorine e6 (Lasephyrin®)		[44,45] lymph node sentinel[46]
	Porficenos[5]	645 nm	Solid tumors [4748]
	Phthalocyanines and naphthalocyanines	670 nm	Melanoma (*in vitro*)[49] Head and neck squamous cell carcinoma, liver cancer (experimental and *in vitro*)[50]
	Phenothiazines[3]	660 nm	Melanomas [51]

Source : Created by the authors with adaptation [7,21.22. 30 - 35]

The second generation of Fs is characterized by purified or synthetic tetrapyrroles, while the third generation refers to purified Fs, now inserted into liposomal carriers and attached to molecules that establish an extra mechanism for targeting the Fs to the tumor tissue. Molecules (pepitides, proteins, polysaccharides, antibody fragments, growth factors, etc.) that have some affinity with certain tumor types are attached to the Fs [22,23].

Based on part of the Warburg effect, which considers that cancer develops in an acidic and anaerobic environment and that even in the presence of oxygen, cancer cells continue to use glycolysis to produce energy, researchers developed a conjugation of chlorine and glucose (G-chlorine) and then chlorine with oligosaccharides (O-chlorine), as the third generation of Fs. These associations increased the intracellular accumulation of Fs by increasing its solubility in water when compared to talaporfin [45,52].

The main disadvantages of first-generation Fs are prolonged photosensitization and low tissue penetration of the activation length in the red

5 These families of Fs have been used more in the antimicrobial modality of PDT, although there have been studies into their antitumor effectiveness.

spectrum, improving somewhat with longer wavelengths. Between 600-800 nm the penetration rate is around 8mm [(2,23)].The second generation, on the other hand, already have improvements in terms of toxicity in the dark and tumor selectivity and they don't stick to the tissues for long [(22,23, 52).]

Most protocols for applying PDT to tumours use intravenous administration of Fs, the undesirable effect of which is prolonged sensitization (for up to weeks)[8,9].For extraosseous lesions in the oral cavity, for example, due to easy access to the tissue, topical applications have been carried out, bypassing the inconvenience of photosensitization[12,19] .

Predominant in the antimicrobial line of PDT but with an effect on neoplastic cells are compounds not derived from the tetrapyrrolic nucleus, characterized as various dyes, especially from the phenitiazine family, especially methylene blue and toluidine blue, as well as derivatives of Nile blue, hypericin, squaraines, curcumin, among others [22].

3.4 Photodynamic therapy (PDT) mediated by protoporphyrin IX - 5-aminolevulinic acid-ALA

5-aminolevulinic acid (5-ALA), most commonly used in oncological PDT for oral and dermatological lesions, is one of the few viable substances for typical application that is already on the market, despite its hydrophilic nature which makes it difficult to penetrate the cell [(23).]

This substance is approved by the *Food and Drug Administration* (FDA) in the United States and by the National Health Surveillance Agency (ANVISA) in Brazil for the treatment of skin lesions such as actinic cheilitis and basal cell carcinoma [24].

5-ALA is a precursor of the Fs endogenous protoporphyrin IX (PpIX), one of the last products of heme group biosynthesis, which occurs in most animal cells [20, 25]. PpIX is a natural porphyrin present in hemoglobin, in the cytochrome c of mitochondria and in other biomolecules. 5-ALA is the first intermediate in the

heme group biosynthesis pathway and is synthesized from glycine succinyl-Coa inside the mitochondria. Outside the mitochondria, two molecules of ALA form porphobilinogen (PBG) and four molecules of PBG form uroporphyrinogen III. The latter is converted into coproporphyrinogen III and, again inside the mitochondria, into protoporphyrinogen IX, which is converted into PpIX by the action of protoporphyrinogen oxidase [16, 23]. As ALA is a precursor of the Fs substance, which is PpIX, it acts on the basis of this activation cascade so that only after the release and irradiation of the Fs does the photodynamic effect begin, which does not occur when other Fs are used[17]
.

Figure 7 schematically shows the conversion of the prodrug 5-ALA to the photosensitizer PpIX.

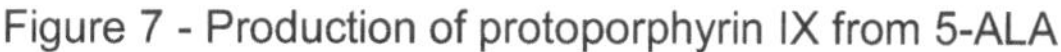
Figure 7 - Production of protoporphyrin IX from 5-ALA

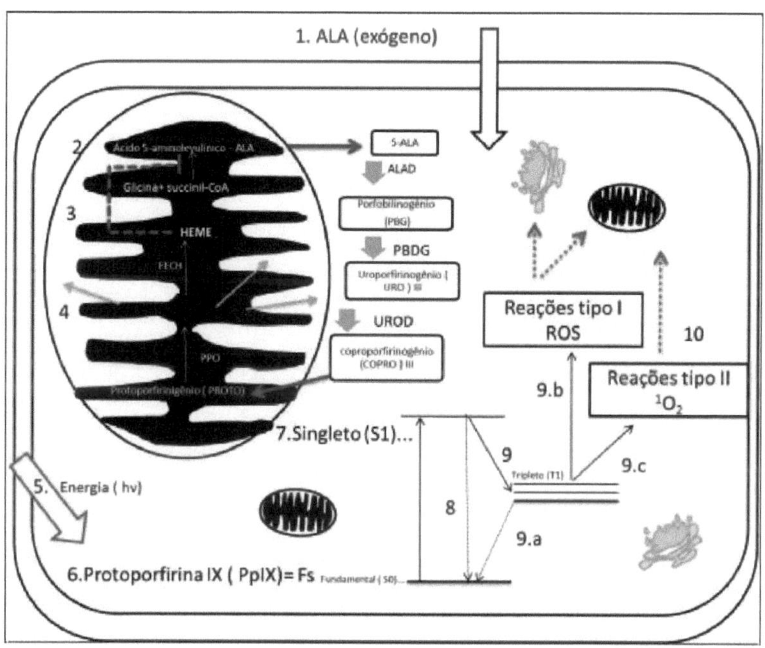

Figure 7- Production of protoporphyrin IX from 5-ALA and diagram of the production of reactive oxygen species in PDT; 1 The penetration of exogenous 5-ALA occurs in a nonselective way into the cells. 2 The synthesis of 5-ALA occurs in the mitochondria and the production of the photosensitizing molecule protoporphyrin IX uses the enzymatic machinery present in heme group biosynthesis. 3 The formation of ALA is tax-dependent on the formation of PpIX and heme groups and is regulated via a negative feed-back control mechanism by free heme groups. 4 Exogenous ALA bypasses the control mechanisms and induces intracellular accumulation of PpIX. 5 In 5-ALA-PDT, after Fs accumulation, irradiation occurs. 6. Fs in the ground state (S^0) absorbs resonant energy (hv). 7. The deposited energy excites Fs in the ground state to the singlet state ($S^{1)}$. 8. The absorbed energy can be released in the form of fluorescence if the Fs returns to the ground state ($S^{0)}$ 9. Excited Fs can also reach the triplet state ($T^{1)}$ from where it can follow a number of paths. 9.a decay back to S^0 9.b react with oxygen by reduction and oxidation reactions and generate free radicals (EROS) - type I reaction. 9.c by energy transfer generate singlet oxygen $^1O_2$- - type II reaction 10. The products of the reactions modify, by oxidative reactions, amino acid residues and unsaturated lipids inside the cell and can lead to its death if it exceeds its antioxidant capacity.

Source : prepared by the authors with adaptation[7,53]

The maximum excitation of the porphyrin occurs in the Soret band (intense absorption band near 400 nm). Tissue penetration at this wavelength is restricted to the superficial layers of tissues. Because of this restriction, irradiations for protoporphyrins have more commonly been done with other excitation sources, located in the red range (620-770 nm) [16,26]. At the cellular level, 5-ALA is taken up in membranes by active transport [20]. Immediately after administration, intracellular PpIX increases rapidly in the first few minutes, peaking at 45 minutes, followed by a slight decrease and saturation around 60-120 minutes in cell culture. The initial localization of PpIX after 5-ALA administration is in the plasma membrane, then perinuclear and finally in the mitochondria after the first hours of 5-ALA incubation [17].The long period of time for the induction of PpIX is due to the hydrophilic properties of 5-ALA, which do not allow it to penetrate the cell membrane easily, and high concentrations of the product are also necessary [16] .

The topical use of ALA has been optimized through mixtures with another pro equivalent drug, methyl aminolevulinate ME-ALA, increasing the production and homogeneity of PpIX with a consequent improvement in the effectiveness of the treatment, an indication that associations present greater advantages than the use of a single drug alone [54].

3.5 Chlorine-mediated photodynamic therapy (PDT)

Chlorine is a natural derivative found in chlorophyll, used pure or as a salt (photoditazine) or in polyvinylpyrrolidone, which are the commercial presentations of laserphyrin and LS11 [22,52]. They absorb in the region between 630-680 nm, allowing treatment of deeper lesions. Foscan® or Temoporfin®, meso-tetra(3-hydroxyphenyl) chlorine or mTHPC, a second generation photosensitizer, is the main commercial representative of this group, which is obtained from the corresponding porphyrin [54, 55].

Studies involving fluorescence microscopy in cell monocultures have shown that mTHPC accumulates in the perinuclear region, endoplasmic reticulum and Golgi apparatus [9,59]. This drug is approved in Europe for the treatment of head and neck neoplasms [56-59]. Mono-L-aspartyl chlorin e6 (NPe6) is also a hydrophilic chlorin derived from chlorophyll, with excellent photosensitizing properties. NPe6 is chemically pure and shows significant absorption at 664 nm. The compound tends to localize in the lysosomal compartments of cell [59]. BPD-MA, Verteporphyrin - a monoacid ring A derivative of Benzoporphyrin - shows rapid absorption, rapid metabolization and is selectively accumulated by endothelial cells [29,59], which is quite significant for tumor vascular damage. This agent has been used in the treatment of age-related macular degeneration [29].

Complex synthetic routes, high production costs and difficulty in purification are some of the factors that have hindered the commercial availability of these compounds [55-58].

3.6 Photodynamic therapy (PDT) mediated by phthalocyanines Synthetic compounds with relatively intense absorption in the region between 630 -680 nm, which have been studied since the 1980s [55], the main representative of this group being silicon phthalocyanine (Pc4), which has been associated with the activation of apoptotic cascades by the extrinsic route, with activation of caspase 8 by increasing the levels of Fas L and Fas , protein complexes which bind to Pro caspase 8 and activate the apoptosis caspase pathway [50].

Immunoexpression of Fas and histological changes suggested apoptosis as a mechanism of cell death in topical FC-Zn PDT [49,57].

3.7 Photodynamic therapy (PDT) mediated by photosensitizers from the phenothiazine family

Phenothiazines are positively charged compounds, which makes them attractive to cell organelles such as mitochondria, but they are dispersed throughout the cytosol until they reach them. The generation of EROS at the mitochondrial site tends to activate apoptosis cascades via the intrinsic or mitochondrial pathway [58].

The most prominent phenothiazine in this group is methylene blue, which has been shown to be effective in terms of cellular phototoxicity against cancer cell lines; however, its effect against mycobacteria in photodynamic therapy is the most studied [23,24,60].

The maximum absorbance of the AM monomer occurs at 664 nm, but in aqueous solution this substance dimerizes and the maximum absorbance occurs at 590 nm, so in aqueous solution at concentrations lower than 20μM there are only monomers. The formation of dimers favors the type I mechanism of PDT [60,61].

Methylene blue for PDT has been effective due to its high quantum yield and high potential for generating singlet oxygen[60]. At a concentration of 10μM of AM associated with 0.5 J /cm ^{2} it is possible to generate subcellular structures indicative of apoptosis, with an increase in the concentration of this Fs, there will be disruption of the plasma membrane leading to cell death by necrosis [61].

Clinical studies with AM in oncology applications have shown total and partial remission (more than fifty percent) of melanomas after five sessions of AM - PDT [51].

3.8 Photodynamic therapy (PDT) mediated by furelenes

Furelenes are spheroidal, nanometric molecules made up only of carbon atoms, fullerene[C60] or simply C60 best represents this category. When photoexcited, C60 passes from the fundamental singlet state ($_1C_{60}$) to the long-lived triplet excited state ($_3C_{60}$)[62], 50-100 μs, which is considered a long time when compared to other Fs [52, 63].

The electronic absorption spectrum of C60 is characterized by several strong absorptions between 190 and 410 nm [64].

The ultra violet absorption peak is a disadvantage due to its low penetration into tissues, but studies indicate that this can be overcome by the chemical connection of one or more structures called red wavelength absorption antennas in the C60 molecule [65]. Temporary alterations to the optical properties of tissues using specific chemical agents, in a procedure called optical cleaning to reduce light scattering, could reduce this inconvenience in the absorption spectrum of furelenes, or any other Fs [66,67].

Two-photon PDT (TP-PDT) has been proposed to expand its medical applications[68], in which two wavelength photons in the near-infrared (NIR) range, instead of a single visible photon, are used to activate Fs, characterizing a way of improving the depth of penetration of the treatment, and may function as an alternative irradiation protocol for better use of this and several other molecules[69].

Furelenes can be chemically modified to achieve the desired lipid affinity and also to improve singlet oxygen production, through a process called functionalization, in which side chains are attached to the molecules. The greatest efficiency of the photodynamic effect, in fact, occurs in functionalized furelenes, but the C60 molecule, when activated, is capable of generating EROS through the type I mechanism. *In vitro* studies have shown the presence of furelenes in membranes and mitochondria using antibodies and indirect immunofluorescence, demonstrating their potential for activating apoptosis and necrosis [70-72].

3.9 Subcellular localization of photosensitizers

The affinity of some Fs for subcellular structures is shown in table 4 [21]Localization preference will determine the pathway of cell death after oxidative stress, as well as contributing to tumor selectivity. Those with affinity for mitochondrial membranes will certainly activate apoptosis cascades, such as Pc4 and benzoporphyrin derivatives, as well as those such as mTHPC chlorin which accumulate in the endoplasmic reticulum. Those that attach to the cell membrane and lysosomes, such as mono-L-aspartyl chlorin e6 (NPe6), will lead the cell to necrosis by altering the potential and consequently rupturing the plasma membrane, or to autophagy through lysosomal activity [21,73,74].

Table 4 - Preferred subcellular location of some photosensitizers

Name/family	**Active ingredient**	**Absorbance peaks**	**subcellular structure**
Photofrin®	Porphyrin (Porifimer sodium)	630-660 nm	Lipid membranes
Photolon®	Chlorine	665 nm	Mitochondria
Foscan® (mTHPC)	m-tetra hydroxyphenylcl	652nm	Mitochondria, reticulum
	orina		endoplasmic , Golgi complex
ALA	5 aminolevulinic acid	635 nm	Cell membranes

Talaporfin sodium (Npe6)	N-aspartyl chlorine e6	664 nm	Lysosomes
Pc4 and FC-Zn	Silicon and zinc phthalocyanine	670 nm	Mitochondria
Phenothiazines	Blueof Methylene	664 nm	Scattered throughout the cytosol and mitochondria
Furelenes	Ceo	190 and 410 nm	Membranes and mitochondria

Source: Created by the authors with adaptation 21,61,72,74

In summary, the peak absorption of tetrapyrrolic photosensitizers such as bacteriochlorines, chlorines and phthalocyanines is concentrated in the red and near-infrared range, where tissue penetration is greatest. Dose fractionation can be more effective than high, single doses. The subcellular location of the photosensitive substance is an important factor in determining the type of cell death, but it is not the only one; the concentration of the Fs and its absorbance must also be taken into account, as well as the energy density of the light source, which also have an influence on this [(21,22)].

Chapter 4 - Mechanisms of proliferation and cell death in PDT

Organelles are the most common subcellular targets for the localization of photosensitizers and the consequent photodynamic effect; however, cytoskeletal structures such as microtubules and microfilaments, as well as cell adhesion components such as desmosomes, have also been described as targets for these substances[26].

The three main mechanisms described after the photodynamic effect are apoptosis, necrosis and autophagy, represented schematically in figure 9. [22]

Figure 9 - Mechanisms of cell death in schematic drawing

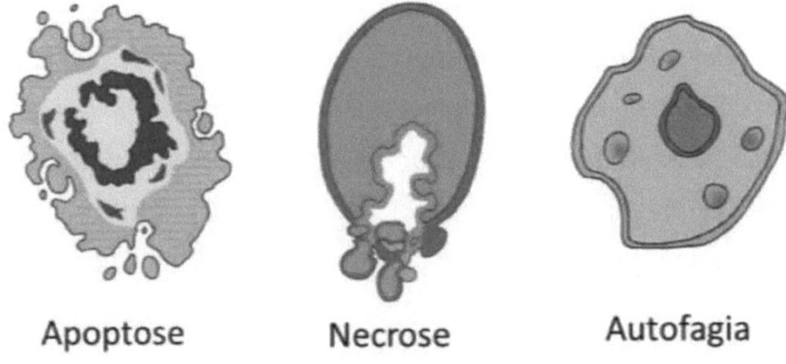

Source : Prepared by the authors

The reactive oxygen species generated from PDT can trigger apoptosis, silent cell death with the formation of apoptotic bodies, necrosis characterized by the rupture of the cell membrane and autophagy initiated in the lysosomes with the formation of intracellular vesicles. [76]

The intense oxidative stress caused by PDT triggers numerous defense and cell death mechanisms. Cell death by the cytotoxic agent can occur through the induction of apoptosis, necrosis, autophagy, inflammatory reactions, immune reactions, as well as damage to the tumor vasculature and healthy surroundings, resulting in the indirect death of the tumor through the induction of hypoxia or starvation. For some photosensitizers, the most important mechanism of therapeutic effect is vascular [21,75-77] .

The mechanisms of cell death and proliferation involved in the photodynamic effect are not yet fully understood. At the same time as clinical studies and research into new technologies for administering PDT, Fs and light sources are progressing, research into basic biological areas is also being carried out with the aim of broadening our understanding of cell behavior in the face of the various PDT modalities [4, 21].

The level of tissue destruction and cytotoxicity after PDT depends on the photosensitizing molecule, its location at the time of irradiation, the total dose administered, the time of exposure to light, the pre-irradiation time, the type of tumour and its oxygenation level. These factors are related to the modulation of the three independent processes that derive from PDT, namely: tumor ischemia through the destruction of support vessels, activation of the immune response and direct tumor destruction, of which some mechanisms will be described below 4, 21,23.

4.1 Apoptosis: Caspase 3 and PDT

Apoptosis is considered to be the most important mechanism of cell death resulting from PDT, especially in oncology, since the imbalance between proliferation and apoptosis is a central topic of discussion in the processes of oncogenesis [21] .

Cells deprived of survival maintenance factors, senescent or damaged cells enter an orderly, non-inflammatory death process called apoptosis [80]. This process leads to the fragmentation of nuclear DNA and the degradation of intracellular structures. Morphologically, it is associated with cell shrinkage and aggregation of organelles (which gives intense eosinophilia under light microscopy), chromatin condensation followed by peripheralization and aggregation of the karyoteca, fragmentation of the nucleus and formation of apoptotic bodies, although there is no fragmentation of the cell membrane [16,37,80,81].

Two main protein families are involved in apoptosis: the Bcl-2 family, which controls the integrity of the mitochondrial membrane, and the caspases, which take part in the cascade of reactions that culminate in the disorganization of the cell nucleus [82].

Apoptosis can be triggered by two routes: either by the binding of death receptors on the plasma membrane (death ligands belonging to the tumor necrosis factor superfamily - **TNF-a**) (known as the extrinsic route), or by the release of pro-apoptotic factors (e.g. cytochrome c) from the mitochondria into the cytosol (intrinsic route). Both pathways trigger the activation of caspases *(cysteine aspartic* acid-specific proteases). These exist in an inactive form (called pro-caspases) and when activated are capable of promoting changes in cell morphology. They can be of the initiator type, formed from the occupation of receptors on the cell membrane (caspases 8, 9 and 10), or effectors (caspases 3, 6 and 7), activated by the initiator caspases and responsible for the destruction of the cell, as they have a short N-terminal domain called DED (death effector domain) which promotes nuclear fragmentation and degradation of the cytoskeleton [82-85].

The *National Council for Cellular Death* (NCCD), in its functional classification of death modalities, points to the activation of caspases 3, 6 and 7 as one of the main biochemical characteristics of apoptosis 8[6]88.

In a review of the mechanisms of cell death generated by PDT, Agostinis *et al.* (2004)[89] point out that this therapy seems to interfere directly with the intrinsic pathway of apoptosis, by promoting an increase in mitochondrial permeability due to the action of EROS, with subsequent release of caspase-activating factors, such as cytochrome c. At the same time, photosensitized cells show a collapse in mitochondrial membrane potential and a drop in ATP in the mitochondria, leading to cell death. At the same time, photosensitized cells exhibit a collapse in mitochondrial membrane potential and a drop in ATP in the mitochondria, leading to death. The authors state that the exact mechanism of how PDT directly contributes to this increase in mitochondrial permeability is not known, but there are indications that this mechanism is linked to the affinity of some mitochondrial membrane proteins to photosensitizing agents, as well as to the sensitivity of the pores to photoxidation, especially to singlet oxygen. This review also describes the activation of pro-apoptotic proteins of the Bcl-2 superfamily (*Bax* and *Bak*), both by EROS and singlet oxygen. When activated, these proteins also trigger an increase in mitochondrial permeability and the release of pro-apoptotic factors. In addition, the action of the EROS generated by PDT activates the *Bax* and *Bak* proteins localized in the endoplasmic reticulum membrane, also increasing the permeability of this organelle, which releases Ca^{2+} into the cytosol. This acts directly on the opening of mitochondrial pores, with consequent release of cytochrome c and activation of caspases. It is also worth mentioning that PDT promotes inhibition of the anti-apoptotic protein Bcl-2, either by Fs or by EROS or by both, also triggering apoptosis [37, 89].

Figure 10 - Hypothetical scheme of the release of pro-apoptotic factors after PDT in apoptosis via the intrinsic pathway

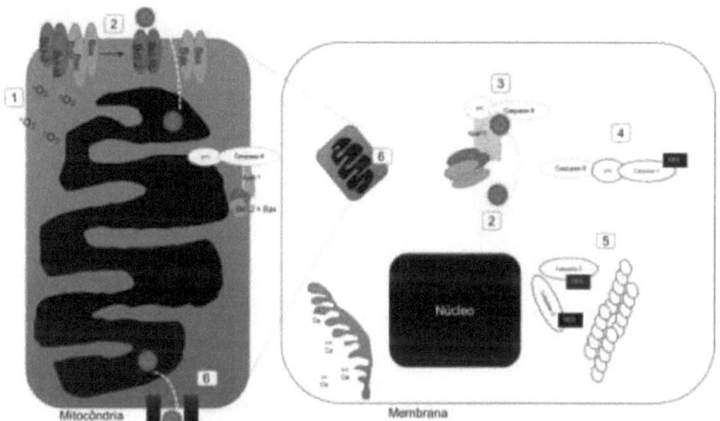

1 Photodynamic effect with release of EROS; 2. Increase in mitochondrial permeability through the Bcl-2 superfamily pores and release of cytochrome c from mitochondria into the cytosol; 3. Apoptosis activating factor 1 - APAF 1 activated and release of initiator caspase 9; 4. Caspase 9 activates effector caspase 3, which has a DED domain. 5) Caspase 3 is activated for nuclear fragmentation and degradation of the cytoskeleton; 6) Alteration of the

membrane potential of the endoplasmic reticulum, release of calcium ions and formation of mitochondrial pores, another route for cytochrome c to leave the cytosol. **Source: prepared by the authors**

The expression of caspase 3 seems to fluctuate depending on the dose of irradiation and the amount of Fs. In a study with a culture of oral squamous cell carcinoma cells treated with PDT mediated by pheophorbide, there was an increase in caspase 3 and other elements indicative of the presence of apoptosis (release of cytochrome c, DNA fragmentation), as well as a decrease in the expression of Bcl-2, shortly after PDT [37].

Another study looked at the expression of caspase 3 in PDT mediated by chlorin Cp6 in oral squamous cell carcinomas induced in hamsters, and found that in the tumors in which the lowest dose of Fs (1.0 mg/kg) was applied, there was no increase in caspase 3. Most of the cells showed a morphological pattern of necrosis. However, when higher concentrations of Fs were used (1.5 mg/kg), there was an increase in caspase 3, indicating activation of this cascade and probably apoptosis[90].

With regard to apoptosis caused by 5-ALA-mediated PDT, several studies involving different cell types (glioma cells, colon carcinoma cells, lymphoma cells) indicate that cell death comes from the mitochondrial pathway, with cytochrome c being released into the cytoplasm. However, the mechanisms of this process are still being debated[91-94].

The apoptosis caused by 5-ALA seems to be linked to the fact that PpIX has an affinity for the peripheral benzodiazepine receptor (PBR), which is part of the mitochondrial membrane. When this receptor is occupied, pores open in the membrane, which favors increased permeability and the release of pro-apoptotic factors, which activate effector caspases[93].

Chen *et al.* (2011) demonstrated that PDT mediated by 5-ALA caused apoptosis of cultured human oral carcinoma cells, which was derived from the activation of the MAPK (*mitogen activation protein kinases*) cascade. In this cascade, apoptosis originated mainly from the activation of the n-terminal JNK kinase and not so much from the p38 kinase and the ERK kinase[94].

The tumor cytotoxicity generated by PDT involves the recruitment of mediators of the apoptosis and necrosis process[78]. One of the effects of PDT on the cell is to destroy the Bcl-2 protein, a protein that regulates the permeability of the mitochondrial membrane[18,15]. PDT also causes selective damage to mitochondria and can initiate a rapid apoptotic response if most of the proteins necessary for the apoptotic cycle are intact, otherwise a necrotic response can occur [12, 17,18, 21].

Another factor that contributes substantially to tumor reduction is the inhibition of angiogenesis[11], since Fs have a predilection for cells with high metabolic activity, such as endotheliocytes[(6)]. Thus, episodes of prolonged ischemia would also be linked to the process of cell death, both through apoptosis and necrosis[79].

The EROS generated during the photodynamic process activate cell signaling cascades that can lead to death by one or more pathways, eliminating altered cells. Because they are very short-lived species, especially singlet oxygen, the action of EROS ends up being restricted to the site where the Fs is located. Thus, Fs that prefer mitochondria lead the cell mainly to apoptosis, while those located in lysosomes or membranes generally signal other pathways such as necrosis and autophagy[34,35].

4.2 Cell proliferation, PCNA and PDT:

Proliferating cell nuclear antigen (PCNA) is a 36kD nuclear protein, a co-factor of DNA polymerase delta, which plays an important role in maintaining genomic stability during DNA replication[95].

DNA damage that delays the replication fork, for example, induces PCNA ubiquitination, activating a bypass of the damaged area in order to prevent the replication forks from collapsing, which could produce broken strands and chromosomal rearrangements. This is why PCNA ubiquitination is a process of strong protein regulation [29]. In the cell cycle, this protein appears in high concentrations in the late G1 and early S phases, and is almost undetectable in cells in the M phase[96].

PCNA immunostaining has been widely used to assess cell proliferation in various tumors and as a cell cycle marker for establishing prognosis [29] .

The kinetics of tumor cells after PDT mediated by systemic Photogem® (sodium porphyrin) and Nd:YAG laser (630 nm, 10 Hz) in a continuous dose was compared to the fractionated dose in a xenotransplant model. The expression of PCNA, understood in the study as a marker of proliferative activity, and VEGF (vascular endothelial growth factor), applied as an indicator of tissue hypoxia in tumors, was analyzed. There was no difference in PCNA levels between 24 hours and 72 hours after PDT when compared to the tumor's baseline levels. There was necrosis only 24 hours after the fractionated dose and an increase in VEGF expression 3 and 6 hours after PDT [97]. Another study also shows an increase in VEGF secretion after systemic PDT in healthy animal brains with the same Fs, but with low energy densities (2J.cm^{-2} and 4J.cm$^{-2)(9)}_{8}$.

Another increase in VEGF levels in the initial 0-6h periods after PDT was observed using hematoporphyrin oligomers and Nd:YAG (630 nm). Tumor necrosis could be seen after 24 hours, but with the presence of remaining neoplastic cells. Damage to tumor vascular cells was investigated using PCNA immunostaining, which was significantly reduced after 24 hours. There was a return to baseline levels in 48 hours due to the remaining tumor cells[99].

Lesions of oral squamous cell carcinoma and oral epithelial dysplasia were treated with PDT mediated by Photofrin® (porfimero sodium - complex mixture of hematoporphyrins) administered systemically and irradiation with an eximer laser (100-200 J/cm$^{2)}$. Biopsies of these lesions taken for histopathological diagnosis were subjected to immunohistochemical analysis for PCNA, VEGF,

CD34 and factor VIII (endothelial cell markers), with the aim of verifying which of these markers could predict the clinical effects of PDT. Only the expression of VEGF was shown to be associated with the clinical results obtained with PDT, in the sense that immunolabeling increased in patients with better clinical results[100,101].

Along the same lines as the previous study, another study evaluated whether the expression of Bak, Mcl-1, caspase 3, caspase-8, caspase-9 (related to apoptosis) p53, p21 or PCNA (related to proliferation) proteins in oral verrucous leukoplakia and hyperplasia could be useful in predicting the clinical results of PDT mediated by typical ALA. Authors carried out an immunohistochemical study of the markers before PDT, compared the groups of patients who showed complete or partial responses to ALA-PDT and concluded that only the ratio between the Bak/Mcl-1 marker indices could be useful as a predictive factor for the clinical efficacy of PDT [102].

The rate of proliferation and apoptosis was demonstrated in keratinocytes from potentially malignant oral lesions, in a carcinogenic line, after three sessions of 5-ALA - PDT, a significant increase in the immunolocalization of caspase and PCNA were identified hours after therapy, with DNA fragmentation detected, however, The authors concluded that there are oscillations between apoptosis and DNA repair in keratinocytes, with a tendency towards repair after 72 hours of ALA-PDT [103].

4.3 Autophagy and BECLIN-1 (BECN-1)

Autophagy (from the Greek "autoingestâo") occurs in all metazoan cells under basal conditions, being a kind of quality control or a mechanism for eliminating cellular waste, as well as a protection mechanism under conditions of cellular stress, mainly nutritional deficiency, hypoxia and oxidative stress[104].Autophagy can be of three types: 1) mediated by chaperones, with protein translocation across the lysosome membrane; 2) microautophagy, which involves the capture of fragments from the cytosol into the lysosomes; 3) and macroautophagy, or classic autophagy, which is characterized by the formation and accumulation of double membrane intermediate vesicles, this being the main and best known mechanism[105].

The autophagy process is subdivided into induction, elongation and maturation stages. A characteristic process of autophagy is the formation of multimembrane organelles initially called phagophores, which elongate and close in on themselves to form autophagosomes or autophagic vacuoles, responsible for loading cytoplasmic waste and taking it to the isosomes [(106)].

Figure 11 - Diagram of cell death by autophagy and participation of the beclin 1 protein

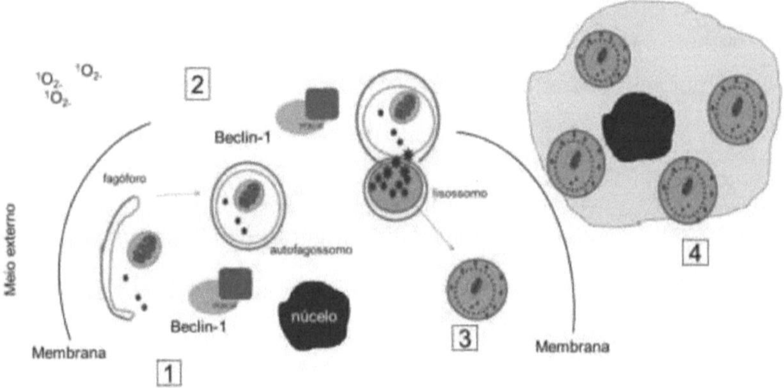

1.BECLIN 1 with PI3-K form a complex that regulates the formation of the phagophore at the beginning of the process (initiation), which sequesters cytoplasmic components as well as organelles and traffics to the lysosomes. 2.Autophagic cytoplasmic degradation requires the formation of a double membrane structure called autophagosome (elongation) 3. Autophagosome - lysosome fusion results in the degradation of cytoplasmic components by lysosomal hydrolases; 4. Excess formation of autophagosomes to eliminate organelles damaged by the oxidative processes of EROS leading the cell to death by autophagy. **Source: prepared by the authors.**

The beclin 1 protein (or BECN1), together with PI3-K (*phosphatidylinositol-3 kinase*) and Atg14 (autophagy protein), forms a complex that regulates the process of nucleation and formation of vesicles, i.e. the formation of the phagophore at the beginning of the process, which can be inhibited by the Bcl-

2, Bcl2/Bcl-XL family (anti-apoptotic proteins) in the absence of a stressful stimulus. Beclin 1 can be considered a marker of autophagy[106,107].

The induction of autophagy by PDT seems to be triggered by EROS and cell death occurs due to the excess formation of autophagosomes to eliminate organelles damaged by oxidative processes. Há studies show that this process, when induced by PDT, is independent of apoptosis and others show that apoptosis and autophagy are concomitant[108]. Bcl-2 inhibits beclin 1, which indicates that by inhibiting apoptosis, the cell also inhibits autophagy. Studies indicate that during PDT, when the photosensitizer is concentrated in the endoplasmic reticulum, beclin 1 is activated and mitophagy is induced, leading to both autophagy and apoptosis. Autophagy is still poorly addressed in basic studies on PDT and oral lesions, and its mechanism has yet to be elucidated [89,108]. However, it seems to play a crucial role in limiting the progression of oral cavity tumors, since its increased expression has been linked to a better prognosis in human epidermoid carcinoma[109] and cystic adenoid carcinoma[110].

In a culture of oral squamous cell carcinoma cells, PDT mediated by pheophorbide a was carried out and high levels of formation of acidic vesicular organelles were observed, suggestive of autophagy, as well as high levels of apoptosis. Autophagy was inhibited, which led to an increase in necrosis rates in the cultures. The authors concluded that PDT mediated by pheophorbide a in oral carcinoma cell cultures is efficient in eliminating tumor cells through apoptosis and that autophagy is present in this process, protecting the cell against necrosis [37].

Another study analyzed the effect of PDT mediated by hexyl 5-ALA on kidney tumors induced in mice. The authors observed high expression of caspase 3 and no change in PCNA. Using transmission electron microscopy, they detected severe damage to the mitochondria, a large number of vacuoles, apoptotic bodies and lipofucsin granules. They concluded that the effect of this type of PDT was mitochondrial apoptosis and autophagy[111].

PDT mediated by 5-ALA was carried out on a culture of pheochromocytoma (PC12) and lung adenocarcinoma (CL10) cells, with the aim of verifying the role of AMPK (*AMP-activated protein kinase*), a protein responsible for establishing cellular homeostasis after severe energy depletion, by inhibiting anabolism and stimulating energy-producing catabolic pathways, as well as stimulating autophagy. The authors found the presence of autophagosomes 2 hours after PDT. The inhibition of autophagy led to a dramatic increase in cell viability. They concluded that autophagy plays a central role in the death mechanism caused by PDT-5-ALA[112].

4.4 Cell necrosis, RIP 1 protein and PDT

Cell death by necrosis has long been characterized as an accidental and pathological process that usually occurs after chemical or physical cell injury, associated with sudden changes in the metabolism and structure of the cell. It is characterized by cell swelling, pyknosis of the nucleus, loss of membrane integrity and extravasation of intracellular components, including enzymes that can be detected in the extracellular medium, such as lactate dehydrogenase and alkaline phosphatase. Há inflammatory response to necrotic tissue, which is basically made up of denatured, coagulated and insoluble proteins[113,114].

Há a type of necrosis that can also occur in a regulated manner, involving a precise sequence of signals, called necroptosis or programmed necrosis [87,115]. This term is used for a type of cell death associated with the activation of the RIP 1 and RIP 3 proteins (members of the RIP family, *receptor integrating protein kinases)* and the morphology of death by autophagy. Necroptosis was first described by Degterev *et al*[116] as a type of death that generally occurs when a cell for some reason is unable to die by apoptosis [113, 114].

The RIP family is made up of seven proteins that have a kinase domain and, among these, RIP 1 is associated with death receptors (belonging to the tumor necrosis factor superfamily - TNF and Fas) and Toll-like receptors that initiate specific cell death cascades[117].When these receptors are occupied, they form a complex with RIP 1 (called complex I) and this undergoes ubiquitination with various molecules associated with death receptors (for example, TRAF2/5, *receptor associated factor 2/5*) and also with anti-apoptotic proteins (such as IAPs, *inhibitor of apoptosis proteins*). This complex activates the NFkB and MAPK pathways[118,119], initiating an anti-apoptosis process. Following the endocytosis of these receptors, this complex is fragmented and RIP1 is deubiquitinated. This forms a second complex (complex II, called DISC, *death-inducing signaling complex*) now with other molecules associated with the TNF-α death receptor (such as TRADD, *TNF-α receptor-associated death domain*, and FADD, *Fas-associated death domain*), as well as with caspase 8. DISC can lead the cell to apoptosis or necrosis. Caspase 8, when activated, promotes the cleavage of RIP 1 and, at the same time, the inhibition of NFkB, favoring apoptosis. However, in situations of high EROS production and energy deficit, in which caspase 8 is inhibited or not formed, RIP 1 does not form complex II and undergoes phosphorylation together with RIP 3, forming a protein complex called the "necroptosome"[119]. It is not yet clear how the necroptosome leads the cell to necrosis, but there are indications that it can cause depolarization of the mitochondrial membrane, an abrupt increase in oxidative stress and an increase in the permeability of the lysosomal membrane and the plasma membrane[117-119]. In addition, one of the effects of the necroptosome is the activation of JNK (*c-Jun NH2-terminal kinase*), which impairs mitochondrial function when high rates of EROS are present in the cell, giving rise to a positive *feedback of* high intracellular production of EROS, leading to necrosis[119]. There may also be cytokine release and Ca^{2+} release into the cytosol, which together interfere with the lipid bilayer of the plasma membrane and the protein integrity of the cytoskeleton [117].

Figure 12 - Diagram of cell death by necrosis of the necroptosis type and participation of RIP family proteins.

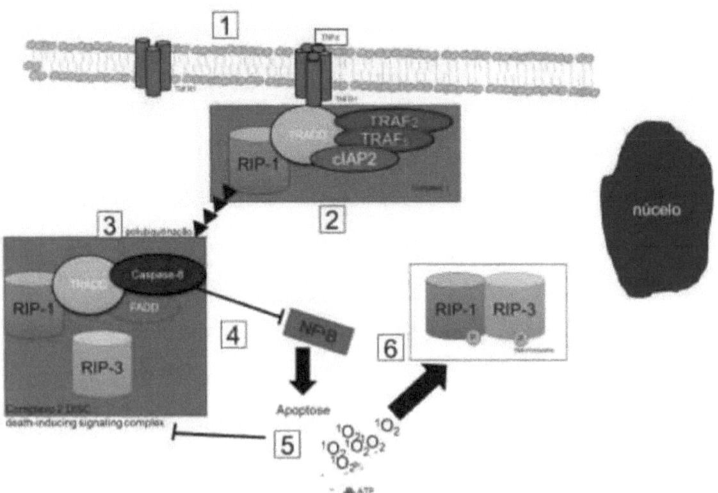

I. occupation of receptors initiating specific cell death cascades 2. formation of complex I; 3. ubiquination of RIP and other molecules associated with death receptors and formation of DISC complex 2. 4. anti-apoptosis 5. high production of EROS and energy deficit RIP 1 does not form complex 2; 6. phosphorylation of RIP 1 and RIP 3, forming the necroptosome which is thought to alter the membrane potential of lysosomes. Source: prepared by the authors

Recently, studies have shown that autophagy contributes to necroptosis. The complex formed by RIP 1 with caspase 8 and the consequent activation of JNK and c-Jun leads to the activation of autophagy. This substantially increases EROS levels, which contributes to irreversible structural changes in the cell. Thus, autophagy together with necroptosis function as a positive *feedback loop,* directing the cell towards death[119].

Some cell culture studies analyzing the expression of RIP 3 are described below.

In a culture of osteosarcoma cells, 5-ALA-mediated PDT was performed on cells deficient in RIP 3 and on cells with normal expression of this protein. Contrary to the hypotheses formulated by the authors, the cells with normal expression of RIP 3 had a higher survival rate after PDT than the deficient cells, as well as greater expression of LC3-II (a marker of autophagosome formation). The authors interpreted the activation of autophagy in efficient RIP

3 cells as a protective effect against the damage caused by PDT, since autophagy, before leading to death, exerts an action of removing defective proteins and organelles, increasing cell survival. The efficient RIP 3 cells also exhibited greater cleavage of caspases 3, 7, 8 and 9 and PARP (poly(ADP-ribose) polymerase) and, therefore, a higher rate of apoptosis. The authors concluded that RIP 3 seems to play an important role in post-PDT apoptosis, and that its presence is essential for activating the caspase pathway. Thus RIP 3, rather than a mediator of necroptosis, would play a protective role by facilitating autophagy and a crucial effect on the establishment of caspase-mediated death[120].

Another study showed that the necrosis induced in cultured glioblastoma cells after 5-ALA-mediated PDT treatment is dependent on the presence of RIP 3, which forms aggregates with RIP 1 after photosensitization. PDT-mediated death was caspase-independent and caused mainly by singlet oxygen. The authors also described low levels of caspase 8 and FADD, proteins present in the formation of complex I and II in TNF-α-stimulated necroptosis. They conclude that the necroptosome formed after PDT may probably have different components to those described so far[121].

Chapter 5- Induction of Potentially Malignant Oral Lesions and Immunolocalization of Cell Death Markers after ALA- PDT

5.1 Oral potentially malignant lesions (OPML) and PDT

PML include a varied group of manifestations, which are white (leukoplakia) or reddish-white (erythroleukoplakia), whose adoption as a clinical diagnosis implies that other diseases with similar clinical signs have been ruled out and which are known not to carry a risk of developing cancer[122].

LPMOs exhibit a wide range of histological features, ranging from mere hyperkeratosis to lesions very close to carcinoma. The risk of malignization of LPMOs is still much debated, with some risk factors linked to this process, such as smoking, alcohol consumption, the presence of dysplasia and recurrence of lesions[123] . There is a consensus that careful clinical follow-up of these lesions is crucial, as well as eradication, especially of those with a histopathological diagnosis of dysplasia[(124).]

Cryosurgery, high-power laser ablation, topical and systemic administration of vitamins and other substances (retinoids, beta carotene, other carotenoids, etc.), as well as PDT are some of the therapeutic modalities proposed for the treatment of LPMO, in addition to conventional surgery[125].

PDT in the management of leukoplakia has shown some efficacy due to its ability to reduce the lesion and its non-invasive nature in the treatment of extensive and superficial areas, generating reduced scarring and low recurrence rates. It also stands out for its high selectivity for cells with increased metabolism, with little or no damage to normal tissue, as well as having no cumulative effect[125-127].

In the context of routine dental practice, topical PDT is particularly more interesting for oral lesions than the systemic modality, since the administration of the Fs does not require isolation of the patient in a light-free environment (this condition is necessary for intravenous administration of the Fs, to minimize the systemic effects generated by photosensitivity). Its execution is also feasible as there are commercial Fs suitable for the wavelengths of the red lasers commonly used in dental practice (660nm, 635 nm among others)[127]. A negative point of typical PDT is the use of Fs that require a long waiting time to reach the ideal peak for irradiation. 5-ALA acid, for example, requires a long interval (1.5 to 3 hours) between the application of the product and irradiation, so that it can penetrate and form the photosensitizing molecule, PpIX. The difficulty lies in keeping the product on the lesion on the oral mucosa without it being dissolved by saliva[128,129].

There are few studies in the literature on the response rates obtained with PDT for LPMO. In the last ten years, clinical findings from around 280 patients have been reported, with satisfactory complete response rates between 25 and 100% and recurrence rates between 0 and 48%[130-134]. Complete clinical remission of LPMOs has been shown from three weekly sessions of PDT mediated by the typical administration of 5-ALA acid[129,132]. However, the interval between sessions and the irradiation protocol, including the fractioning or not of the parameters, are still highly debatable.

5.2 Proposition

To establish the anatomical-chronological relationship of cell death markers present after 5-ALA-mediated PDT in chemically-induced PML.

a) To establish the percentage of lesion reduction as a function of the experimental times of 6h, 24h, 48h and 72 hours after PDT application.

b) Check the immunohistochemical expression of PCNA, caspase 3, beclin 1 and RIP 1 proteins in each of these periods.

c) Determine the time interval after PDT in which cell death predominates.

d) Suggest the time interval between PDT sessions based on the expression of the markers studied.

5.3 Material and method

Some of the results and discussion of the study entitled: Analysis of the expression of cell death markers in potentially malignant oral lesions induced with 4-NQO and treated with photodynamic therapy, which relates ALA- PDT to the expression of cell proliferation nuclear antigen- PCNA and some cell death markers, namely caspase 3, beclin and RIP 1, as well as their immunolabeling pattern in potentially malignant leukoplakic lesions induced in rat tongues, the method of which will be briefly described.

The procedures described below were previously approved by the Ethics Committee for the Use of Animals (CEUA) of the Institute of Biomedical Sciences of the University of São Paulo (ICB-USP) (certificate no. 157) (Appendix A).Prior to the design of the sample groups, an experiment was carried out to characterize the induction model with 4-NQO, in which weekly histopathological analysis of the lingual mucosa was carried out. This experiment was set up to check the tissue changes caused by the carcinogen over time, in order to see if a period of up to 16 weeks was sufficient to induce dysplastic lesions comparable to those described in the literature, taking into account the local conditions of the vivarium and the type/age of the animal. At the same time, biochemical and hematological tests were carried out to determine the degree of systemic toxicity of 4-NQO [135].

A. Experimental groups

Eighty-four male Wistar rats weighing around 200g were randomly divided into:

a) <u>PDT Group</u> - Composed of 42 animals, in which LPMO was induced by the typical application of 4-NQO solution and then treated with PDT.

b) <u>Positive control group</u> - Composed of 32 animals in which LPMO was induced by topical application of 4-NQO solution, but without PDT treatment.

c) <u>Negative control group:</u> composed of 10 animals submitted to the same experimental conditions, but without induction of lesions and without PDT treatment.

The experimental times at which euthanasia took place were 6, 24, 48 and 72 hours after PDT (8 animals for each period). After 72 hours of PDT, another 10 animals underwent a second PDT cycle, five of which were euthanized 6 hours after this second treatment and another five after 72 hours.

The Central Bioterium of the Biomedical Sciences Institute of the University of São Paulo provided the animals, which were fed commercial food (Labina®, Purina, Bayer, Brazil) and water *ad libitum*, subjected to 12-hour light-dark cycles and kept in individual cages throughout the experiment.

B. Induction of potentially malignant lesions with 4-NQO

4-nitroquinoline-oxide (4-NQO) (Sigma, Aldrich, USA) was diluted in propylene glycol at a concentration of 5mg/ml and applied to the lingual mucosa (back and belly) of the animals using a microbrush, three times a week, for 16 weeks[136,138].

The amount of solution used in each application was around 0.15 mg, calculated by weighing the material in the microbrush. The entire procedure for handling the carcinogen was carried out strictly following the biosafety precautions recommended by the manufacturer, with the use of two gloves, anti-gas masks, goggles and a white apron covered with a disposable apron. Residues of the solution, as well as all the material used and contaminated, were sent for incineration. The animals were isolated in the vivarium in individual shelves. Induction was interrupted the week before PDT.

C. Injury monitoring

After 16 weeks of applying 4-NQO, the volume of the tongue and the induced lesions were measured using a pachymeter. Only lesions with a diameter greater than or equal to 5 mm were selected to be treated with PDT. Tongue volume was calculated by multiplying thickness X distance from one lateral edge to the other X distance from the apex to the base, obtaining a value in mm^3. The size of the lesions was determined by measuring their largest diameter (in mm). In the case of multiple lesions, only the largest lesion was measured. Measurements were taken immediately before PDT and at the time of euthanasia, in order to compare the effects of the treatment on the tongue as a whole and on the size of the lesions. Only one operator performed the measurements blindly. These data have been previously published.[135]

D. PDT protocol

To perform PDT, the animal was previously anesthetized with intraperitoneal injections of ketamine (0.1ml/g) and xylazine (0.01ml/g). After confirming deep sedation, a solution of 5-ALA (Sigma Aldrich, Saint Louis, USA) at a concentration of 20% in EDTA and physiological solution homogenized with lanolin and Vaseline Kquida[139] was applied topically to the site of the lesion. The ALA was kept on the mucosal surface for 2 hours and renewed every 30 minutes, followed by irradiation[(140)]. The output power of the laser was checked using a power meter (Power max 600 -Molectron- USA). To confirm the presence of a greater amount of PpIX in the PDT group compared to the controls, a fluorescence test was carried out for PpIX. The data from this test can be found in Appendix B, which shows a higher level of fluorescence in the samples with 5-ALA.

Irradiation was carried out with a diode laser (660nm, MM Optics, Sâo Carlos, Brazil), with the parameters described below (table 5). The area of the irradiated point corresponded to the area of the laser spot[141].

Table 5- Parameters of the PDT activation source

Wavelength -Λ- (nm)	660
Power (mW)	40
Energy (J/point)	3,6
Energy density per point (J/cm^2)	90

Area of the point (cm^2)	0,04
Time per point (min)	1,5
No. of irradiations	1
No. of irradiated points	2
Power density mW/cm^2	1000

The second PDT cycle was carried out using the same protocol after 72 hours for a group of 10 animals.

The animals in the control groups underwent anesthesia and were kept in similar conditions to the PDT group.

E. Euthanasia and removal of material for analysis

The animals in the PDT group were euthanized in a CO_2 chamber at 6h, 24h, 48h and 72h after PDT in the first session, and at 6h and 72h in the second session. The control groups (positive and negative) underwent euthanasia in the period coinciding with 72 hours after PDT. The tongue was then removed, sectioned longitudinally with one half frozen and the other fixed in 20% paraformaldehyde in anhydrous monobasic sodium phosphate buffer solution pH 7.0, always prepared on the same day as use and the fragments were sent for histological processing.

F. Histopathological analysis

The material was fixed for a minimum of 24 hours and a maximum of 48 hours, after which it was sectioned in the median sagittal plane and processed for paraffin embedding. Firstly, two 10-minute baths were made in the formaldehyde buffer solution (anhydrous monobasic sodium dibasic phosphate) and then, to start dehydrating the tissue, the pieces were immersed in increasing amounts of ethanol (from 30% ethanol lasting 10 minutes to 70% ethanol). They were then introduced into an automatic histological processor (Leica 1010, Germany) to continue the increasing chain of ethanol baths up to absolute ethanol. They were then bathed in 50% ethanol/xylol, two baths in xylol and, finally, immersed in paraffin with a melting point of 60°C, making the tissue blocks. Cuts measuring 3µm were obtained on a microtome and then automatically stained in hematoxylin and eosin using a staining machine (Sakura Finetek, USA Inc.) and analyzed under conventional light microscopy.

In order to establish the cellular morphological changes after PDT in the epithelium of the lingual mucosa (ventral side), two examiners read the slides blindly, observing the following elements: degree of hyperkeratosis, hyperplasia of the basal layer, atrophy, loss of polarity of the basal layer cells, cellular vacuolization, nuclear hyperchromatism, loss of cellular cohesion and inflammation in the connective tissue. These elements were graded subjectively by prior calibration between the two examiners, and classified as: 0 - absent; 1 - discreet (less than 25% of the field showing the alteration); 2 - moderate (between 25% and 75% of the field showing the alteration); 3 - intense (more than 75% of the field showing the alteration). The regions of interest were analyzed at 100X and 400X magnification. These results were previously published [135].

Three additional histological sections of the same specimen were obtained, stained in H&E and submitted to morphometry. The epithelial area (keratin and other layers) was quantified in four successive fields (400X magnification) by manual delineation using the appropriate tool in the Image J 111 software. Using the same method, the area of keratin alone was quantified in all groups. The entire procedure was carried out by a single blind operator.[135]

G. Immunohistochemical analysis

The streptavidin-biotin method was used for the immunohistochemical study with the anti-caspase3, anti-RIP 1, anti- beclin-1 and anti-PCNA antibodies. The protocols used for each antibody are described in Table 6.

Chart 6 - Protocols used in immunohistochemistry reactions

Antibody	Clone	Titration	Incubation period	Pre-treatment	Antibody control
Anti-caspase3 Abcam Inc	Monoclonal (E87)	1:50	1h	Water bath 95°C, 40min citric acid buffer *pH* 6.0, 0.01M	Carcinoma of the uterine cervix
Anti-RIP 1 (H-207) Santa Cruz Biotechnology Inc	Polyclonal	1:25	1h	Water bath 97°C, 45min citric acid buffer, *pH* 6.0, 0.01M	Small intestine
Anti Beclin 1 Abcam Inc	Polyclonal	1:50	1h	Water bath 95°C, 40min citric acid buffer, *pH* 6, 0.01M	Brain
Dako Anti-PCNA	Monoclonal (PC10)	1:100	1 h	Water bath 95°C, 30min citric acid buffer, *pH* 6.0, 0.01M	Oral squamous cell carcinoma

In order to obtain quantitative data on immunohistochemical expression, a manual counting method was used to evaluate the percentage of positive cells in a universe of 1000 cells per sample. The cells considered positive for PCNA, beclin 1 and RIP 1 were those that showed clear nuclear marking, and these nuclei were quantified. As the caspase3 marking was predominantly cytoplasmic, the criterion adopted was to quantify only those cells

in which the nuclei were visible and the cell periphery was clearly marked. If these criteria were not met, the cell was considered negative. Counting was carried out at 400X magnification, using a zoom of up to 200X and the manual particle counting tool in the Image J software[142]. In all counts, the intensity of the marking was not taken into account. The entire procedure was carried out by a single blind operator.

H. Statistical analysis

Descriptive statistics were used using the mean and standard deviation for the numerical data obtained from the tongue/lesion measurements, the area of the epithelium and the percentages obtained from the quantification of the cells. For the intensity data of the elements present in the histopathological analysis, the median and minimum and maximum values were adopted. The Kruskal-Wallis test was used for multiple comparisons and the Mann-Whitney non-parametric test for two-by-two analyses. The significance level adopted was 5%.

5.4 Results

The results regarding the induction of leukoplakic lesions, the clinical and histopathological evaluation of the linguas treated with ALA- PDT have been previously published and are described in references 135,103.

A. Clinical and histological aspects of lesions induced and treated with PDT.

After 16 weeks of typical application of 4-NQO, the ventral and dorsal surfaces of the tongue showed hyperkeratotic white plaque, sometimes with undefined boundaries (Figure 13).

Figure 13 - Chemically induced oral leukoplakia lesions

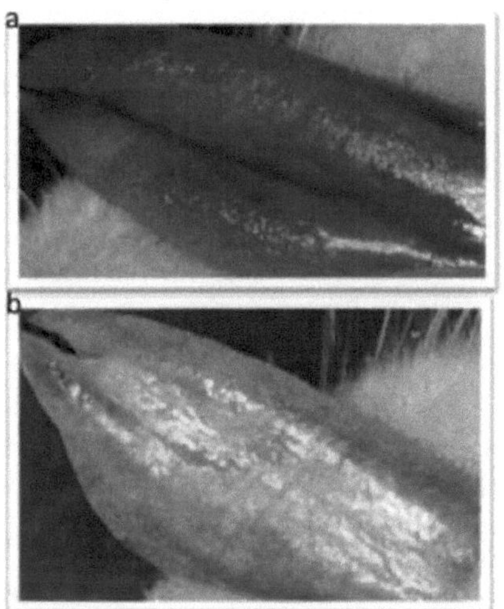

Figure 13 - Clinical appearance of lesions induced with 4-NQO on the lingual mucosa of rats. a. Initial appearance. b: Hyperkeratotic white plaque after 16 weeks of induction: Initial appearance. b: White hyperkeratotic plaque after 16 weeks of **induction.** Source: research results.[6]

Lesions measuring 5mm or more were treated with PDT and, at the time of euthanasia, the linear measurement of the lesions and the volume of the tongue were obtained and compared with the measurements taken before treatment. In this study, it was also observed that there was a significant reduction (in the order of 50%) in the largest diameter of the lesion in the second PDT cycle, both at 6h and 72h, compared to all the experimental periods of the first cycle. In the first cycle, there was no significant reduction in the lesion between the periods and in relation to the positive control[135]. The clinical appearance after ALA-PDT is shown in figure 14.

Figure 14 - Clinical and histological appearance of induced LOPM treated with PDT

---

6 Other images and descriptions in Barcessat et al 135

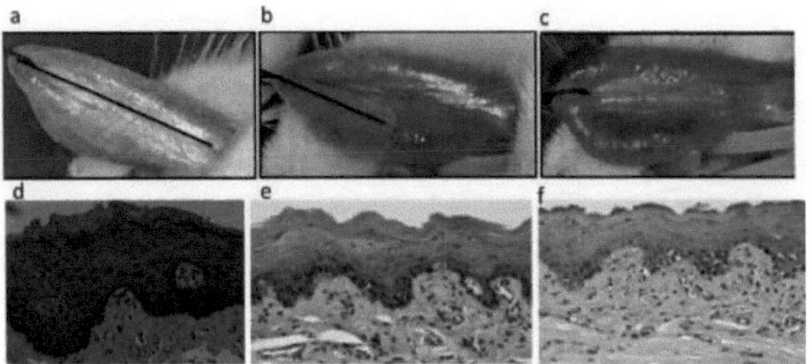

Figure 14 - shows a potentially malignant oral lesion induced by 4-NQO (a) treated with ALA- PDT after 24 (b) and 72 (c) hours after PDT, in which the clinical reduction of the leukoplakic area can be seen. Histologically, the appearance of an induced lesion (d), the effect of PDT after 24 (e) and 72 hours (f) which, although not from the same sample, are compatible with the clinical aspects. **Source: research results.**

Experimental induction with 4-NQO causes the formation of cellular atypia in the epithelium of the lingual mucosa, with a predominance of nuclear hyperchromatism, inversion of polarity of the basal layer, drop-like projections, hyperkeratosis and areas of epithelial atrophy[135].

In general, the 6h and 24h periods after PDT showed greater intensity of basal layer hyperplasia, loss of basal layer cell polarity and nuclear hyperchromatism than the other PDT periods.

B. Descriptive analysis of immunohistochemical expression

2.1 PCNA

Immunohistochemical tests with PCNA in tongue dysplastic lesions treated with ALA- PDT and their respective controls, using the method described above, show nuclear expression of the cells located predominantly in the basal layer and with varying intensity. In the untreated negative control, PCNA expression is restricted to the basal layer of the epithelium, with some positive nuclei interspersed with negative ones. In the positive control, the intensity of labeling becomes more pronounced, and a greater number of positive nuclei are visible. In the epithelia treated with PDT, especially in the first 6 hours, there is intense labeling of the nuclei in the basal layer, which is hyperplasticized, as well as some nuclei in the upper layers. [103] After 72 hours of PDT, PCNA expression is much lower than in the other groups. Other results including the TUNEL test for cell death and analysis of a second PDT cycle are shown in reference 103[103].

Figure 15 - PCNA immunolocalization after ALA-PDT

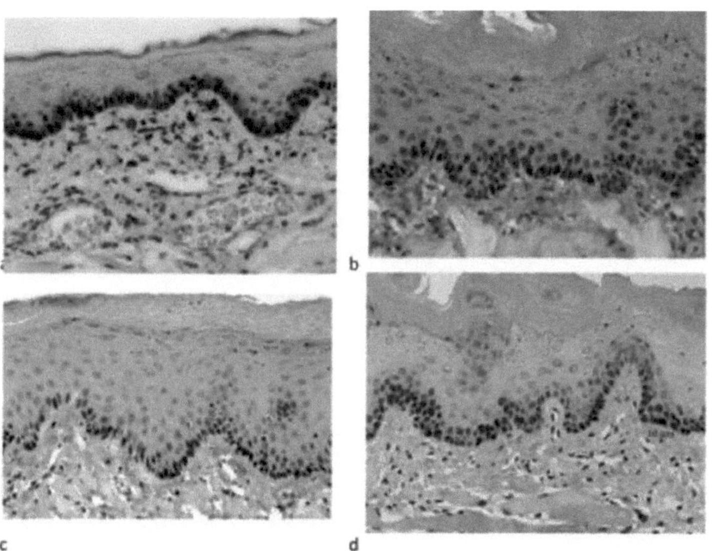

Figure 15 - Immunohistochemical expression of PCNA in epithelium after 16 weeks of chemical carcinogenesis (a), after 6 (b) 24 (c) and 72 (d) hours of ALA-PDT (Streptavidin-biotin, 400X). Scale = 50µm. See description in the text above. **Source : Research results**

2.2 Caspase - 3

The immunohistochemical expression of caspase 3 was generally cytoplasmic with a diffuse pattern in all the groups and periods analyzed, being restricted to the basal and suprabasal layers of the epithelium. There was greater intensity in the groups treated with PDT, especially at 6 hours. During these periods, it was possible to visualize the concentration of immunohistochemical expression in the cell periphery, delimiting the cells (figure 16).

Figure 16 - Caspase immunolocalization after ALA-PDT

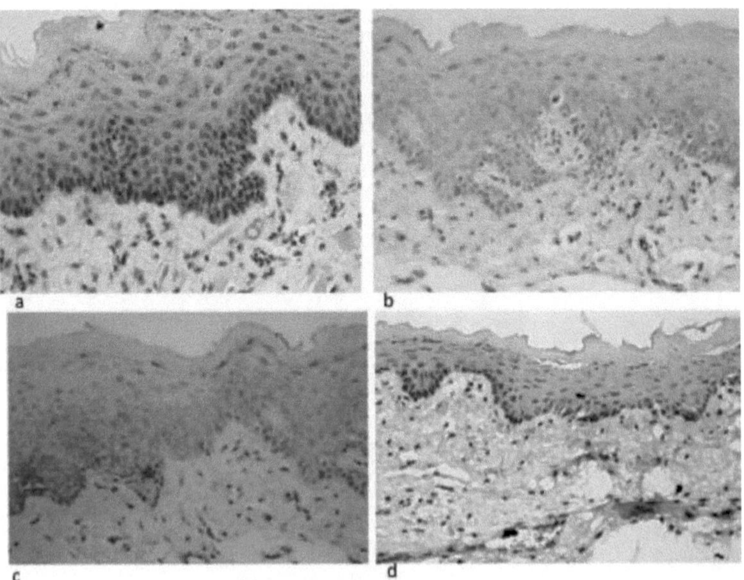

Figure 16 - Immunohistochemical expression of caspase 3 in epithelium after 16 weeks of chemical carcinogenesis (a), after 6 (b) 24 (c) and 72 (d) hours of ALA- PDT (Streptavidin-biotin, 400X). Scale = 50μm. See description in the text above.

Source: Survey results

2.3 Beclin - 1 and RIP-1

The immunohistochemical expression of beclin 1 showed a granular pattern in the cytoplasm of the basal layer cells and a homogeneous pattern, with varying intensity, in the cell nuclei of the superficial layers (Figure 17) . Apparently, the experimental period of 6 hours after PDT showed greater intensity, mainly because there were more cells with positive cytoplasm. The positive control showed several nuclei in the superficial layers positive for the protein, and some cells in the basal layer with positivity in the cytoplasm, but several cells in this layer did not show the marking. After 72 hours of PDT, there was a reduction in the intensity of expression.

For the study described, the immunohistochemical expression of RIP 1 was also cytoplasmic in the basal layer and nuclear in the upper layers. The positive control showed discrete labeling, mainly in the basal layer. In 6h PDT, there was an increase in the intensity of labeling compared to the positive control. In the 6h periods, the nuclear pattern extends more frequently to the upper layers than in the other groups and periods. In PDT 24h and PDT 72h, nuclear marking was absent or very discreet (Figure 18) .

Figure 17 - Immunolocalization of the BECLIN - 1 protein after ALA-PDT

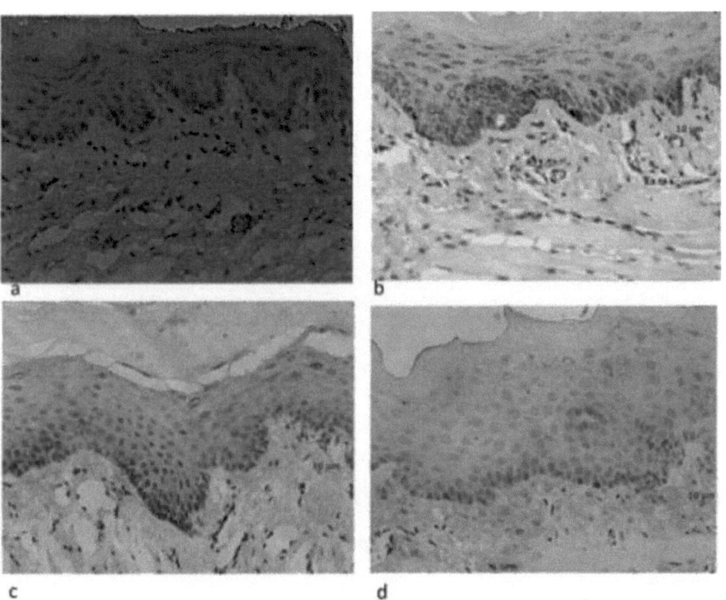

Figure 17- Immunohistochemical expression of beclin 1 in epithelium after 16 weeks of chemical carcinogenesis (a), after 6 (b) 24 (c) and 72 (d) hours of ALA- PDT (Streptavidin-biotin, 400X). **Source: research results**

Figure 18 - Immunolocalization of the RIP 1 protein after ALA-PDT

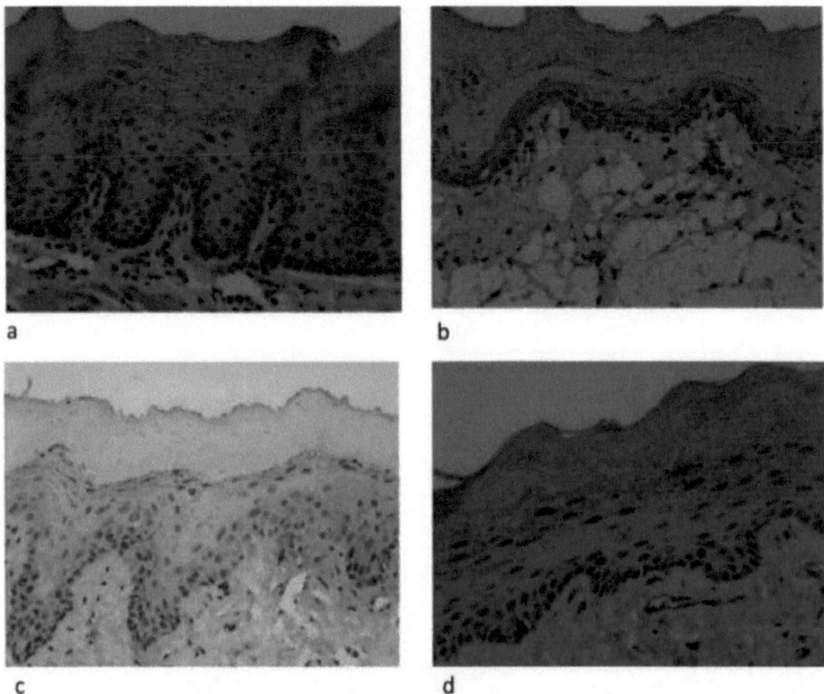

Figure 18 - Immunohistochemical expression of RIP 1 in the different groups and experimental periods (Streptavidin-biotin, 400X). Scale = 50μm. See description in the text.**Source: research results**

C. Analysis of epithelial cells positive for each of the proteins analyzed

Graph 1 shows the average percentage of positive epithelial cells for each of the proteins analyzed. Considering the controls, the highest frequency of positive cells was for PCNA, with significant differences in relation to the other markers for both the negative control (Kruskal-Wallis test, p=0.0002) and the positive control (Kruskal-Wallis test, p=0.0019). In the PDT group of the first cycle, the percentage of positivity for caspase 3 was statistically higher than all the other proteins in the 6-hour period (PCNA - p=0.0294; beclin 1 - p=0.0034; RIP 1 - p=0.0285); in the 24-hour period, there was a significant predominance of caspase 3 compared to beclin 1 (p=0.0106) and RIP 1 (p=0.0285), but not in relation to PCNA. At 48 hours, there were no differences between the proteins; at 72 hours, PCNA was significantly more expressed in relation to beclin 1 (p=0.0472) and RIP 1 (p=0.0090), but not in relation to caspase 3 (p=0.6015). In the second PDT cycle, at 6h and 72h there was a substantial increase in the percentage of PCNA-positive cells, which was significant in relation to all the other proteins (p=0.0090 for all crosses); during this period, the percentage of caspase 3 was significantly higher than that of beclin 1 (p=0.0107 for 6h and 72h) and RIP 1 (p=0.0090 for 6h and 72h), and there were no differences between these two. The drop in expression of beclin 1 and RIP 1 at 72h compared to 6h stands out, which was not observed for caspase 3 and PCNA.

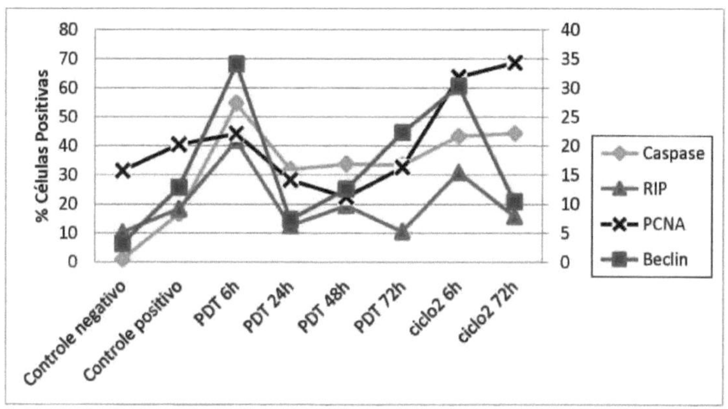

Graph 1 - Mean percentage (±standard deviation) of epithelial cells positive for PCNA caspase 3, beclin 1 and RIP 1 in the different groups and experimental periods.

5.5 - Discussion

The purpose of this study was to analyze, in anatomical and chronological terms, the immunohistochemical expression of PCNA, caspase 3, beclin 1 and RIP 1 in LPMO treated with PDT mediated by 5-ALA. The aim of this analysis was to understand how these markers are expressed over time after PDT, in order to suggest the key period in which there could be a possible recovery of the epithelium. This was understood to be represented by the high expression of PCNA and the low expression of the other markers. The importance of this analysis, apart from the fact that it potentially contributes to understanding the mechanism of 5-ALA-mediated PDT, also lies in the possibility of being able to modify or prove the interval between PDT sessions, which are already carried out empirically in the clinic.

The PDT protocol adopted caused clinical changes that suggest the beginning of a process of remission of the induced lesions, which was clinically visible.

There was a significant reduction in the lesion of around 50% in the second PDT session, which indicates the need for more than one session to understand the therapeutic effectiveness of this protocol[103].

The only obvious clinical sign of the action of the first PDT session on the lesions was an increase in tongue volume at 6h and 24h[103,135]. This was probably due to the intense interstitial edema caused by the vasodilation caused by the therapy. However, in this initial session, especially 6 hours after irradiation, cellular morphological changes were already observed in the epithelium which modified the atypia induced by 4-NQO. Hyperplasia of the basal layer, nuclear hyperchromatism and cell vacuolization may indicate high proliferation accompanied by cell degeneration. It is worth noting that there was no increase in the degree of cellular atypia, nor was there any greater indication of malignancy, although tests have not been carried out with other markers that are more suitable for verifying malignancy in dysplastic lesions.

The result of these transformations instituted by PDT in the present study seems to be epithelial atrophy, as evidenced by the significant reduction in epithelial thickness in the 6h PDT and in the periods of the second PDT cycle[103]. However, the recovery of this thickness still seems to be very efficient, since the other periods of the first cycle (from 24 to 72 hours) show epithelia with a similar size and sometimes larger than the positive control. In fact, the still high expression of PCNA may contribute to supporting this statement, which will be discussed further below. Thus, based on these morphological results, we can infer that the PDT protocol adopted led to changes in the kinetics of maintaining epithelial thickness, as well as being efficient in starting to reduce lesions from the second cycle onwards, but did not generate the necrosis and intense epithelial atrophy described in clinical studies of oral squamous cell carcinomas treated with PDT. It could therefore be considered that the fluence adopted or the irradiation time may have been low, causing a sublethal effect or only apoptosis in the cells. On the other hand, there are indications that there is a relationship between the clinical aspect of the lesion and the efficacy of PDT mediated by 5-ALA; however, a TUNEL test applied to the same specimens showed a high rate of cell death[103]. A clinical study of oral verrucous hyperplasia showed that 3 to 4 sessions of PDT (LED-635-nm, 100 mW/cm^2 100 J/cm^2) were required for the total remission of lesions up to 1.5 cm, and that orthokeratinized lesions may require more sessions[144]. It is likely that the lesions induced in this study, which ranged from 8 to 14mm in size, also follow the rule described for oral verrucous hyperplasia, together with the fact that they are also hyperkeratinized.

The descriptive analysis of the immunohistochemistry showed changes in the marking pattern of the antigens studied at the experimental PDT times in relation to the negative and positive controls. In general, there was an increase in the intensity of expression and extension to the suprabasal and spinous layers after PDT, especially at 6 hours. This was partially confirmed by the significant differences observed in the count of positive cells, as described below.

The significant increase in PCNA-positive cells 6 hours after PDT, and even more so 6 hours into the second cycle, can be interpreted not so much as an increase in cell proliferation, but rather as the establishment of a process to maintain genomic stability[95] in the face of the intense aggression caused by excessive ROS. As PCNA is found in large quantities in the late G1 phase and in the S phase, cell division is not confirmed by this marker, but it can be said that the protein and DNA corrections necessary for proliferation have been triggered. This must probably be occurring in viable cells, given that the thickness of the epithelium was the same as the positive control in the second cycle, even though there was a drastic reduction 6 hours after PDT in the first cycle. This result partially agrees with that described by Uehara et al. 1999 in xenotransplantation of oral squamous cell carcinoma, in which an increase in the percentage of PCNA-positive cells was also detected, but this occurred between 48 and 72 hours after PDT. These discrepancies are probably due to differences in the proliferation kinetics of tumors and dysplastic lesions, as well as differences in the PDT protocol. In other studies on PCNA and PDT in oral squamous cell carcinoma, there were no differences in the amount of expression of PCNA-positive cells between the control and experimental periods after PDT, either for 5-ALA-mediated PDT[145] or Photofrin®-mediated PDT[97]. Thus, there is some agreement in assuming that viable dysplastic cells after PDT do not lose their ability to proliferate, a fact which may explain the recurrences after PDT in various tumors.

The increase in PCNA expression was accompanied by a high percentage of caspase 3 positive cells in this study. There was a peak in caspase 3 expression 6 hours after PDT, which showed a significant reduction in the other periods, but was still higher than the positive control. As caspase 3 is activated at the end of the apoptosis cascade, and because an antibody was used that marks cleaved and therefore active caspase 3, it can be inferred that there was probably a high level of apoptosis during this period. In the second cycle, the percentage of cells was also high, but did not reach the levels observed in 6 hours of the first cycle. The trend towards an increase in caspase 3 observed in the first cycle coincides with several studies in the literature using different PDT techniques and oral squamous cell carcinoma cells or tissue [37,90,95,99].

Thus, this study confirmed the trend already described in the literature that apoptosis seems to predominate after PDT in techniques that do not induce much necrosis.

As with caspase 3, the percentage of cells positive for beclin 1 was also significantly higher after 6 hours of PDT, indicating that proteins involved in autophagy were activated, more precisely with the formation of the phagophore at a time coinciding with caspase 3. This result is similar to another described in the literature using cultured oral squamous cell carcinoma cells, which were treated with PDT mediated by pheophorbide1 [37], and in studies with PDT mediated by 5-ALA in other tumors[111, 112] . The concomitant activation of apoptosis and autophagy has recently been discussed in the literature[108] , and there is a tendency to believe that both processes can be activated simultaneously, and that autophagy-related proteins also participate in caspase-mediated cell death.

The percentage of cells positive for RIP 1 was also higher at 6h after PDT, also indicating a triggering of the necroptosis pathway by PDT, generally at times coinciding with the increase in expression of the other markers. One study had already shown an increase in the expression of RIP-3 in glioblastoma cell cultures treated with PDT mediated by 5-ALA (0.5mM ALA, 3h incubation, 2.3Jcm^{-2}), as well as a high level of necrosis[119]. However, no necrosis was observed in the tissues analyzed, not even microscopically, which suggests that the increased expression of RIP 1 is probably much more related to apoptosis and autophagy than to necrosis. In fact, in another study using PDT mediated by 5-ALA (1mM ALA, 3h incubation, 20.61J/cm^2) on osteosarcoma cells, carried out by the same group of authors as the previous study[120], the importance of RIP-3 in activating caspases and forming autophagosomes was proven, even more so than in causing necrosis. These differences between the two studies are probably due to discrepancies in sensitivity to PDT between the two cell types (glioblastoma cells and osteosarcoma cells), as well as variations in the PDT technique. Thus, it can be interpreted that PDT mediated by 5-ALA led to significant expression of RIP 1 shortly after its introduction, and that this expression is probably more linked to apoptosis and autophagy than to necrosis.

In the concomitant analysis of the markers, it can be seen that at 6 hours after PDT there was a significant predominance of cells expressing caspase 3 in relation to the other proteins, which allows us to infer that at this time there was a predominance of apoptosis over possible DNA repair and cell proliferation mechanisms. It is worth mentioning that the 6-hour interval after irradiation established in this study was arbitrary, based on another study which showed that there was no expression of caspase 3 and PCNA in the first three hours after irradiation[130].

On the other hand, it can be said that from 24 to 72 hours this apoptosis effect is attenuated, and that DNA corrections now prevail with a view to cell cycle progression, since there is a significant reduction in all death-related markers and a significantly higher number of PCNA-positive cells. There seems to be a tendency for genomic corrections to be more exacerbated from the second cycle onwards, even outweighing the apoptosis rates and PCNA rates observed[103]. In this sense, it can be said that the cells express proteins of protection and genomic correction in a different way to that observed in the first cycle, a fact that may be linked to possible mechanisms of resistance to PDT. Further studies are needed to clarify this trend towards greater

PCNA expression in a second PDT cycle.

Among the periods analyzed, the most significant period of return to epithelial renewal seems to be 72 hours after PDT. There was no difference between the caspase 3 and PCNA indices during this period, but there was between this marker and RIP 1 and beclin 1. It is worth noting that PCNA expression was still lower than that of the positive control, which may indicate that PDT, despite the rapid damage caused by singlet oxygen, activates other cascades and has a delayed effect on the cells. However, this effect is much more attenuated than at the start of the process. It can therefore be said that it is not recommended to extend the duration of a second PDT session by more than 72 hours. Due to the drop in expression of all the markers 24 hours after PDT, it could also be suggested that the ideal period for this second dose would be 24 hours after the first, adding the pro-apoptotic effects instituted in 6 hours during this period of protein depletion. Some studies, albeit with different protocols, have already followed this 24-hour interval between PDT sessions for oral squamous cell carcinoma, with systemic porphyrin [97, 101] and for oral verrucous hyperplasia, with ALA [146, 147], which seems to have a positive effect on lesion remission.

In summary, the present study showed that PDT mediated by 5-ALA caused an increase in the expression of caspase 3, beclin 1 and RIP 1 in LPMO in the first 6 hours after therapy. In this PDT model, these proteins seem to interact in death mechanisms by apoptosis and autophagy, but not by necrosis. For the clinical condition created in this study, the ideal interval for the next session is 24 hours and the critical interval for intense cell recovery is 72 hours.

6. Final considerations

PDT mediated by 5-ALA, applied topically to induced LPMO, was able to generate a significant reduction in lesions (in the order of 50%).

The increase in the expression of beclin 1 and RIP 1 accompanied that of caspase 3, indicating that there is a predominance of apoptosis and autophagy, but not necrosis, in the cell death processes induced by PDT.

The increase in the percentage of cells positive for caspase 3, beclin1, RIP 1 and PCNA occurred mainly 6 hours after PDT, with a significant decrease in this positivity occurring 24 hours after PDT.

Based on the findings of cell kinetics in the PML after therapy, a 24-hour interval between PDT sessions is considered the most appropriate, without extending beyond 72 hours.

For cancer therapy, there should be a more detailed discussion of the inflammatory effect after therapy and the stimulation of immune function, obviously taking into account the type and location of the tumor.

References[7]

1. Buchholz J, Kaser-Hotz B. Combined photodynamic therapy and hyperthermia with water-filtered infrared light for the treatment of cutaneous squamous cell carcinoma in 15 cats: A pilot study. Kleintierpraxis. 2010;55(5):248-254.

2. Dougherty TJ, Marcus SL. Photodynamic therapy. Eur J Cancer. 1992;28A(10):1734-1742.

3. Biel MA. Photodynamic therapy treatment of early oral and laryngeal cancers.Photochem Photobiol. 2007;83(5):1063-1068.

4. Kessel D. Adventures in photodynamic therapy: 1976-2008. J Porphyr Phthalocyanines. 2008;12(8):877-880.

5. Machado AED. Photodynamic therapy: Principles, potential of application and perspectives. Quimica Nova. 2000;23(2):237-243.

6. Krosl G, Korbelik M, Krosl J, Dougherty GJ. Potentiation of photodynamic therapy-elicited antitumor response by localized treatment with granulocytemacrophage colony-stimulating factor. Cancer Res. 1996;56(14):3281-3286.

7. Wen X, Li Y, Hamblin MR. Photodynamic therapy in dermatology beyond non-melanoma cancer: an update. Photodiagnosis Photodyn Ther. 2017 pii: S1572-1000(17)30235-1.

8. Sharma SK, Mroz P, Dai T, Huang YY, St Denis TG, Hamblin MR. Photodynamic Therapy for Cancer and for Infections: What Is the Difference? Isr J Chem. 2012 ;52(8-9):691-705.

9. Agostinis P, Berg K, Cengel KA, Foster TH, Girotti AW, Gollnick SO, Hahn SM, Hamblin MR, Juzeniene A, Kessel D, Korbelik M, Moan J, Mroz P, Nowis D, Piette J, Wilson BC, Golab J. Photodynamic therapy of cancer: an update.

7 Vancouver style

CA Cancer J Clin. 2011;61(4):250-81.

10. Tamietti BF, Machado AH, Maftoum-Costa M, Da Silva NS, Tedesco AC, Pacheco-Soares C. Analysis of mitochondrial activity related to cell death after PDT with AlPCS(4). Photomed Laser Surg. 2007 Jun;25(3):175-179.

11. Castano AP, Mroz P, Hamblin MR. Photodynamic therapy and anti-tumour immunity.Nat Rev Cancer. 2006;6(7):535-545.

12. Nowis D, Makowski M, Stoklosa T, Legat M, Issat T, Golab J. Direct tumor damage mechanisms of photodynamic therapy. Acta Biochim Pol. 2005;52(2):339-352.

13. Garg AD, Nowis D, Golab J, Agostinis P. Photodynamic therapy: illuminating the road from cell death towards anti-tumour immunity. Apoptosis. 2010 Sep;15(9):1050-1071.

14. Nowis D, Legat M, Grzela T, Niderla J, Wilczek E, Wilczynski GM, Glodkowska E,Mrówka P, Issat T, Dulak J, Józkowicz A, Was H, Adamek M, Wrzosek A, Nazarewski S, Makowski M, Stoklosa T, Jakóbisiak M, Golab J. Heme oxygenase-1 protects tumor cells against photodynamic therapy-mediated cytotoxicity. Oncogene. 2006;25(24):3365-74.

15. Allison RR. PDT frontiers. Photodiagnosis Photodyn Ther.2009;6(2):135-136.

16. Kessel D, Oleinick NL. Photodynamic therapy and cell death pathways. Methods Mol Biol. 2010;635:35-46.

17. Maftoum-Costa M, Naves KT, Oliveira AL, Tedesco AC, da Silva NS, Pacheco-Soares C. Mitochondria, endoplasmic reticulum and actin filament behavior after PDT with chloroaluminum phthalocyanine liposomal in HeLa cells. Cell Biol Int. 2008;32(8):1024-8.

18. Buytaert E, Dewaele M, Agostinis P. Molecular effectors of multiple cell death pathways initiated by photodynamic therapy. Biochim Biophys Acta. 2007;1776(1):86-107.

19. Mitton D, Ackroyd R. A brief overview of photodynamic therapy in Europe. Photodiagnosis Photodyn Ther. 2008;5(2):103-11.

20. Detty MR, Gibson SL, Wagner SJ. Current clinical and preclinical photosensitizers for use in photodynamic therapy. J Med Chem. 2004;47(16):3897-3915. Review.

21. Corrêa L, Barcessat ARP, Photodynamic therapy in the treatment of malignant and potentially malignant oral lesions. In: PDT: Antimicrobial photodynamic therapy in dentistry.1. Rio de Janeiro : Elsevier; 2015. 271 - 286

22. Abrahamse H, Hamblin MR. New photosensitizers for photodynamic therapy. Biochem J. 2016;473(4):347-64.

23. Stapleton M, Rodes LE: Photosensitizers for photodynamic therapy of cutaneous disease. J Dermatol Treat 2003; 14: 107.

24. Allison RR, Sibata CH. Oncologic photodynamic therapy photosensitizers: a clinical review. Photodiagnosis Photodyn Ther. 2010; 7:61-75.

25. Oliveira, C.S.; Turchiello, R.; Kowaltowski, A.J.; Indig, G.L.; Baptista, M.S. Major determinants of photoinduced cell death: Subcellular localization versus photosensitization efficiency. Free Radic. Biol. Med. 2011; 51:824833.

26. van Straten D, Mashayekhi V, de Bruijn HS, Oliveira S, Robinson DJ. Oncologic Photodynamic Therapy: Basic Principles, Current Clinical Status and Future Directions. Cancers (Basel). 2017 Feb 18;9(2). pii: E19.

27. Ribeiro JN, Flores AV, Mesquita R, Nicola JH, Nicola EM. Photodynamic therapy: a light in the fight against cancer. Physicae. 2005; 5(2):5.

28. Torezan L, Niwa AB, Neto CF. [Photodynamic therapy in dermatology: basic principles]. An Bras Dermatol. 2009;84(5):445-59.

29. P.G. Calzavara-Pinton, M. Venturini, R. Sala. Photodynamic therapy: update 2006 - Part , J. Eur. Acad dermatol Venereol. 2007, 21, 293-302

30. Saavedra R, Rocha LB, Dabrowski JM, Arnaut LG. Modulation of

biodistribution, pharmacokinetics, and photosensitivity with the delivery vehicle of a bacteriochlorin photosensitizer for photodynamic therapy. ChemMedChem. 2014; 9:390-398.

31. Gross S, Gilead A, Scherz A, Neeman M, Salomon Y. Monitoring photodynamic therapy of solid tumors online by BOLD-contrast MRI. Nat Med. 2003; 9:1327-1331.

32. Kharkwal GB, Sharma SK, Huang YY, Dai T, Hamblin MR. Photodynamic therapy for infections: clinical applications. Lasers Surg Med. 2011 Sep;43(7):755-67.

33. Morley S, Griffiths J, Philips G, Moseley H, O'Grady C, Mellish K, Lankester CL, Faris B, Young RJ, Brown SB, Rhodes LE. Phase IIa randomized, placebo-controlled study of antimicrobial photodynamic therapy in bacterially colonized, chronic leg ulcers and diabetic foot ulcers: a new approach to antimicrobial therapy. Br J Dermatol.2013; 168:617-624.

34. Verma S, Sallum UW, Athar H, Rosenblum L, Foley JW, Hasan T. Antimicrobial photodynamic efficacy of side-chain functionalized benzo[a]phenothiazinium dyes. Photochem Photobiol. 2009 Jan-Feb;85(1):111-8.

35. Kamkaew A, Lim SH, Lee HB, Kiew LV, Chung LY, Burgess K. BODIPY dyes in photodynamic therapy. Chem Soc Rev. 2013; 42:77-88.

36. Wen X, Li Y, Hamblin MR. Photodynamic therapy in dermatology beyond non-melanoma cancer: an update. Photodiagnosis Photodyn Ther. 2017 Jun 21.

37. Ahn MY, Yoon HE, Kwon SM, Lee J, Min SK, Kim YC, Ahn SG, Yoon JH. Synthesized Pheophorbide a-mediated photodynamic therapy induced apoptosis and autophagy in human oral squamous carcinoma cells. J Oral Pathol Med. 2013 Jan;42(1):17-25.

38. Bourré L, Rousset N, Thibaut S, Eléouet S, Lajat Y, Patrice T. PDT effects

of m-THPC and ALA, phototoxicity and apoptosis. Apoptosis. 2002 Jun;7(3):221-30.

39. Beardsley RM, McCannel CA, McCannel TA. Recurrent leakage after Visudyne photodynamic therapy for the treatment of circumscribed choroidal hemangioma.Ophthalmic Surg Lasers Imaging Retina. 2013 May-Jun;44(3):248-51.

40. Shimada K, Matsuda S, Jinno H, Kameyama N, Konno T, Arai T, Ishihara K,Kitagawa Y. The Noninvasive Treatment for Sentinel Lymph Node Metastasis by Photodynamic Therapy Using Phospholipid Polymer as a Nanotransporter of Verteporfin. Biomed Res Int. 2017;2017:7412865.

41. Kvaal SI, Warloe T. Photodynamic treatment of oral lesions. J Environ Pathol Toxicol Oncol. 2007;26(2):127-33. Review.

42. Kulyk O, Ibbotson SH, Moseley H, Valentine RM, Samuel ID. Development of a handheld fluorescence imaging device to investigate the characteristics of protoporphyrin IX fluorescence in healthy and diseased skin. Photodiagnosis Photodyn Ther. 2015 Dec;12(4):630-9.

43. Basset-Seguin N. [PDT panoramic view. Principle, photosensitizers, light sources and validated indications in dermatology]. Ann Dermatol Venereol.

2013 Nov;140 Suppl 2:223-8.

44. Nakamura T, Oinuma T. Usefulness of Photodynamic Diagnosis and Therapy using Talaporfin Sodium for an Advanced-aged Patient with Inoperable Gastric Cancer (a secondary publication). Laser Ther. 2014 Sep 30;23(3):201-10.

45. Kataoka H, Nishie H, Hayashi N, Tanaka M, Nomoto A, Yano S, Joh T. New photodynamic therapy with next-generation photosensitizers. Ann Transl Med. 2017 Apr;5(8):183.

46. Nishida T, Takeno S, Nakashima K, Kariya M, Inatsu H, Kitamura K, Nanashima A. Salvage photodynamic therapy accompanied by extended

lymphadenectomy for advanced esophageal carcinoma: A case report. Int J Surg Case Rep. 2017;36:155-160.

47. Abels C. Targeting of the vascular system of solid tumors by photodynamic therapy (PDT). Photochem Photobiol Sci. 2004 Aug;3(8):765- 71.

48. tockert JC, Canete M, Juarranz A, Villanueva A, Horobin RW, Borrell JI, Teixidó J, Nonell S. Porphycenes: facts and prospects in photodynamic therapy of cancer. Curr Med Chem. 2007;14(9):997-1026. Review.

49. Freitas LF, Hamblin MR, Anzengruber F, Perussi JR, Ribeiro AO, Martins VCA,Plepis AMG. Zinc phthalocyanines attached to gold nanorods for simultaneous hyperthermic and photodynamic therapies against melanoma in vitro. J Photochem Photobiol B. 2017 Aug;173:181-186.

50. Manoto SL, Houreld N, Hodgkinson N, Abrahamse H. Modes of Cell Death Induced by Photodynamic Therapy Using Zinc Phthalocyanine in Lung Cancer Cells Grown as a Monolayer and Three-Dimensional Multicellular Spheroids. Molecules. 2017 May 16;22(5).

51. Tardivo JP, Del Giglio A, Paschoal LH, Ito AS, Baptista MS. Treatment of melanoma lesions using methylene blue and RL50 light source. Photodiagnosis Photodyn Ther. 2004 Dec;1(4):345-6. doi: 10.1016/S1572-1000(05)00005-0.

52. St Denis TG, Hamblin MR. Synthesis, bioanalysis and biodistribution of photosensitizer conjugates for photodynamic therapy. Bioanalysis. 2013 May;5(9):1099-114.

53. Barcessat ARP, Analysis of the expression of cell death markers in potentially malignant oral lesions induced with 4-NQO and treated with photodynamic therapy. (Doctoral Thesis).Sâo Paulo: School of Dentistry, University of Sâo Paulo ; 2013.

54. Fujita AK, Rodrigues PG, Requena MB, Escobar A, da Rocha RW, Nardi AB, Kurachi C, de Menezes PF, Bagnato VS. Fluorescence evaluations for

porphyrin formation during topical PDT using ALA and methyl-ALA mixtures in pig skin models.Photodiagnosis Photodyn Ther. 2016 Sep;15:236-44.

55. De Oliveira K. T, de Souza J M, Gobo N R S, de Assis F F,Brocksom T J.Basic Concepts and Applications of Porphyrins, Chlorins and Phthalocyanines as Photosensitizers in Photonic Therapies. Rev. Virtual Quim. 2015 2015; 7(1): 310-335.

56. Brown SB, Brown EA, Walker I., The Present and Future Role of Photodynamic Therapy in Cancer Treatment. Lancet Oncol, 5, 497-508, 2004.

57. Almeida RD, Manadas BJ, Carvalho AP, Duarte CB. Intracellular signaling mechanisms in photodynamic therapy. Biochim Biophys Acta. 2004 Sep 20;1704(2):59-86.

58. Teiten MH, Bezdetnaya L, Morlière P, Santus R, Guillemin F. Endoplasmic reticulum and Golgi apparatus are the preferential sites of Foscan localization in cultured tumour cells. Br J Cancer. 2003 Jan 13;88(1):146-52.

59. Teiten MH, Marchal S, D'Hallewin MA, Guillemin F, Bezdetnaya L. Primary photodamage sites and mitochondrial events after Foscan photosensitization of MCF-7 human breast cancer cells. Photochem Photobiol. 2003 Jul;78(1):9-14.

60. Mellish KJ, Cox RD, Vernon DI, Griffiths J, Brown SB. In vitro photodynamic activity of a series of methylene blue analogues. Photochem Photobiol. 2002 Apr;75(4):392-7.

61. Gabrielli, DS. Photodynamic efficiency of phenothiazines in mitochondria and tumor cells (Master's thesis). Sâo Paulo: Instituto de Quimica, Universidade de Sâo Paulo, 2007.doi:10.11606/D.46.2007.tde- 18102007-153851. Accessed on: 2017-08-17.

62. Santos, LJ, Rocha, GP, Alves, RB, Freitas RP. Fullerene[C60]: chemistry and applications. Chem. Nova [online]. 2010, vol.33, n.3

63. Agostinis P, Berg K, Cengel KA, Foster TH, Girotti AW, Gollnick SO, Hahn

SM, Hamblin MR, Juzeniene A, Kessel D, Korbelik M, Moan J, Mroz P, Nowis D, Piette J, Wilson BC, Golab J. Photodynamic therapy of cancer: an update. CA Cancer J Clin. 2011;61(4):250-81.14

64. Imahori, H.; Umeyama, T. In Fullerenes Principles and Apllications; Langa, F.; Nierengarten, J.-F., eds.; The Royal Society of Chemistry: Cambridge, 2008, ch. 9.

65. J. Baffreau, S. Leroy-Lhez, N. Vân Anh, R. M. Williams, and P. Hudhomme, Fullerene C60-Perylene-3, 4:9, 10-bis (dicarboximide) lightharvesting dyads: Spacer-length and bay-substituent effects on intramolecular.

66. Tuchin VV, Wang RK, Yeh AT. Optical clearing of tissues and cells. J Biomed Opt. 2008 Mar-Apr;13(2):021101.

67. Hirshburg J, Choi B, Nelson JS, Yeh AT. Correlation between collagen solubility and skin optical clearing using sugars. Lasers Surg Med. 2007 Feb;39(2):140-4.

68. Gu B, Wu W, Xu G, Feng G, Yin F, Chong PHJ, Qu J, Yong KT, Liu B. Precise Two-Photon Photodynamic Therapy using an Efficient Photosensitizer with Aggregation-Induced Emission Characteristics. Adv Mater. 2017 Jul;29(28).

69. Sun B, Wang L, Li Q, He PP, Liu H, Wang H, Yang Y, Li J. Bis(pyrene) Doped Cationic Dipeptide Nanoparticles for Two-Photon-Activated Photodynamic Therapy.Biomacromolecules. 2017 Aug 14

70. Mroz P, Pawlak A, Satti M, Lee H, Wharton T, Gali H, Sarna T, Hamblin MR.Functionalized fullerenes mediate photodynamic killing of cancer cells: Type I versus Type II photochemical mechanism.Free Radic. Biol. Med.43, 711(2007).

71. Sperandio FF, Sharma SK, Wang M, Jeon S, Huang YY, Dai T, Nayka S, de Sousa SC, Chiang LY, Hamblin MR. Photoinduced electron-transfer

mechanisms for radical-enhanced photodynamic therapy mediated by watersoluble decacationic C_{70} and C_8^ Fullerene Derivatives. Nanomedicine. 2013 May;9(4):570-9.

72. Huang YY, Sharma SK, Yin R, Agrawal T, Chiang LY, Hamblin MR. Functionalized fullerenes in photodynamic therapy. J Biomed Nanotechnol. 2014 Sep;10(9):1918-36.Review.

73. Luksiene Z, Eggen I, Moan J, Nesland JM, Peng Q. Evaluation of protoporphyrin IX production, phototoxicity and cell death pathway induced by hexylester of 5-aminolevulinic acid in Reh and HPB-ALL cells. Cancer Lett. 2001 .

74. Kramer-Marek G, Serpa C, Szurko A. Spectroscopic Properties and Photodynamic Effects of New Lipophilic Porphyrin Derivatives: Efficacy, Localization and Cell Death Pathways. J. Photochem, Photobiol. B: Biol, 84(1), 1-14, 2006

75. Usuda J, Kato H, Okunaka T. Photodynamic Therapy (PDT) for Lung Cancers. Journal of Thoracic Oncology, 1(5), 489-493, 2006

76. TRIESSCHEIJN M., BAAS P., SCHELLENS J. H. M. et al, Photodynamic Therapy in Oncology. Oncologist, 11, 1034-1044, 2006

77. Firczuk M, Nowis D, Go⅛b J. PDT-induced inflammatory and host responses. Photochem Photobiol Sci. 2011 May;10(5):653-63.

78. Huang YY, Vecchio D, Avci P, Yin R, Garcia-Diaz M, Hamblin MR. Melanoma resistance to photodynamic therapy: new insights. Biol Chem. 2013 Feb 1;394(2):239-50.

79. Reeves KJ, Reed MW, Brown NJ. The role of nitric oxide in the treatment of tumors with aminolaevulinic acid-induced photodynamic therapy. J Photochem Photobiol B. 2010 Dec 2;101(3):224-32.

80. Martin SJ. Getting the measure of apoptosis. Methods. 2008 Mar;44(3):197-9

81. Almeida RD, Manadas BJ, Carvalho AP, Duarte CB. Intracellular signaling mechanisms in photodynamic therapy. Biochim Biophys Acta. 2004 20;1704(2):59-86..

82. Moor AC. Signaling pathways in cell death and survival after photodynamic therapy. J Photochem Photobiol B. 2000 Aug;57(1):1-13..

83. Logue SE, Martin SJ. Caspase activation cascades in apoptosis. Biochem Soc Trans. 2008 Feb;36(Pt 1):1-9.

84. Morgan J, Potter WR, Oseroff AR. Comparison of photodynamic targets in a carcinoma cell line and its mitochondrial DNA-deficient derivative. Photochem Photobiol. 2000;71(6):747-57.

85. Creagh EM, Conroy H, Martin SJ. Caspase-activation pathways in apoptosis and immunity. Immunol Rev. 2003;193:10-21. Review.

86. Galluzzi L, Vitale I, Abrams JM, Alnemri ES, Baehrecke EH, Blagosklonny MV,Dawson TM, Dawson VL, El-Deiry WS, Fulda S, Gottlieb E, Green DR, Hengartner MO, Kepp O, Knight RA, Kumar S, Lipton SA, Lu X, Madeo F, Malorni W, Mehlen P, Nunez G, Peter ME, Piacentini M, Rubinsztein DC, Shi Y, Simon HU, Vandenabeele P, White E, Yuan J, Zhivotovsky B, Melino G, Kroemer G. Molecular definitions of cell death subroutines: recommendations of the Nomenclature Committee on Cell Death 2012. Cell Death Differ. 2012;19(1):107-20.

87. Kroemer G, Galluzzi L, Vandenabeele P, Abrams J, Alnemri ES, Baehrecke EH,Blagosklonny MV, El-Deiry WS, Golstein P, Green DR, Hengartner M, Knight RA, Kumar S, Lipton SA, Malorni W, Nunez G, Peter ME, Tschopp J, Yuan J, Piacentini M, Zhivotovsky B, Melino G; Nomenclature Committee on Cell Death 2009. Classification of cell death: recommendations of the Nomenclature Committee on Cell Death 2009. Cell Death Differ. 2009;16(1):3-11.

88. Galluzzi L, Maiuri MC, Vitale I, Zischka H, Castedo M, Zitvogel L, Kroemer

G. Cell death modalities: classification and pathophysiological implications. Cell Death Differ. 2007 Jul;14(7):1237-43.

89. Agostinis P, Buytaert E, Breyssens H, Hendrickx N. Regulatory pathways in photodynamic therapy induced apoptosis. Photochem Photobiol Sci. 2004 g;3(8):721-9.

90. Dube A, Sharma S, Gupta PK. Evaluation of chlorin p6 for photodynamic treatment of squamous cell carcinoma in the hamster cheek pouch model. Oral Oncol. 2006;42(1):77-82.

91. Inoue K, Karashima T, Kamada M, Shuin T, Kurabayashi A, Furihata M, Fujita H, Utsumi K, Sasaki J. Regulation of 5-aminolevulinic acid-mediated protoporphyrin IX accumulation in human urothelial carcinomas. Pathobiology. 2009;76(6):303-14.

92. Furre IE, MOller MT, Shahzidi S, Nesland JM, Peng Q. Involvement of both caspase-dependent and -independent pathways in apoptotic induction by hexaminolevulinate-mediated photodynamic therapy in human lymphoma cells.Apoptosis. 2006;11(11):2031-2042.

93. Oleinick NL, Morris RL, Belichenko I. The role of apoptosis in response to photodynamic therapy: what, where, why, and how. Photochem Photobiol Sci. 2002;1(1):1-21.

94. Chen HM, Liu CM, Yang H, Chou HY, Chiang CP, Kuo MY. 5-aminolevulinic acid induces apoptosis via NF-κB/JNK pathway in human oral cancer Ca9-22 cells. J Oral Pathol Med. 2011 Jul;40(6):483-489.

95. Chen J, Bozza W, Zhuang Z. Ubiquitination of PCNA and its essential role in eukaryotic translesion synthesis. Cell Biochem Biophys. 2011;60(1-2):47- 60

96. Naryzhny SN. Proliferating cell nuclear antigen: a proteomics view. Cell Mol Life Sci. 2008;65(23):3789-3808.

97. Togashi H, Uehara M, Ikeda H, Inokuchi T. Fractionated photodynamic therapy for a human oral squamous cell carcinoma xenograft. Oral Oncol.

2006;42(5):526-532.

98. Zhang X, Jiang F, Zhang ZG, Kalkanis SN, Hong X, deCarvalho AC, Chen J, Yang H, Robin AM, Chopp M. Low-dose photodynamic therapy increases endothelial cell proliferation and VEGF expression in nude mouse brain. Lasers Med Sci. 2005;20(2):74-79

99. Uehara M, Inokuchi T, Sano K, ZuoLin W. Expression of vascular endothelial growth factor in mouse tumors subjected to photodynamic therapy. Eur J Cancer.2001;37(16):2111-2115.

100. Uehara M, Ikeda H, Nonaka M, Sumita Y, Nanashima A, Nonaka T, Asahina I.Predictive factor for photodynamic therapy effects on oral squamous cell carcinoma and oral epithelial dysplasia. Arch Oral Biol. 2011;56(11):1366-1372.

101. Uehara M, Inokuchi T, Sano K, Sekine J, Ikeda H. Cell kinetics of mouse tumor subjected to photodynamic therapy--evaluation by proliferating cell nuclear antigen immunohistochemistry. Oral Oncol. 1999;35(1):93-97.

102. Yu CH, Chen HM, Lin HP, Chiang CP. Expression of Bak and Bak/Mcl-1 ratio can predict photodynamic therapy outcome for oral verrucous hyperplasia and leukoplakia. J Oral Pathol Med. 2013 Mar;42(3):257-262.

103. Barcessat AR, Huang I, Rosin FP, dos Santos Pinto D Jr, Maria Zezell D, Corrêa L. Effect of topical 5-ALA mediated photodynamic therapy on proliferation index of keratinocytes in 4-NQO-induced potentially malignant oral lesions. J Photochem Photobiol B. 2013 5;126:33-41.

104. Ganley IG, Lam du H, Wang J, Ding X, Chen S, Jiang X. ULK1.ATG13.FIP200 complex mediates mTOR signaling and is essential for autophagy. J Biol Chem. 2009 1;284(18):297-305.

105. Itman BJ, Rathmell JC. Metabolic stress in autophagy and cell death pathways.Cold Spring Harb Perspect Biol. 2012 1;4(9):a008763.

106. Elgendy M, Sheridan C, Brumatti G, Martin SJ. Oncogenic Ras-induced

expression of Noxa and Beclin 1 promotes autophagic cell death and limits clonogenic survival. Mol Cell. 2011; 8;42(1):23-35.

107. Salminen A, Kaarniranta K, Kauppinen A. Beclin 1 interactome controls the crosstalk between apoptosis, autophagy and inflammasome activation: Impact on the aging process. Ageing Res Rev. 2012 7;12(2):520-534.

108. Buytaert E, Callewaert G, Vandenheede JR, Agostinis P. Deficiency in apoptotic effectors Bax and Bak reveals an autophagic cell death pathway initiated by photodamage to the endoplasmic reticulum. Autophagy. 2006 Jul-;2(3):238-40.

109. Kapoor V, Paliwal D, Baskar Singh S, Mohanti BK, Das SN. Deregulation of Beclin 1 in patients with tobacco-related oral squamous cell carcinoma. Biochem Biophys Res Commun. 2012; 15;422(4):764-9.

110. Liang LZ, Ma B, Liang YJ, Liu HC, Zheng GS, Zhang TH, Chu M, Xu PP, Su YX,Liao GQ. High expression of the autophagy gene Beclin 1 is associated with favorable prognosis for salivary gland adenoid cystic carcinoma. J Oral Pathol Med. 2012;41(8):621-9.

111. Arum CJ, Gederaas OA, Larsen EL, Randeberg LL, Hjelde A, Krokan HE, Svaasand LO, Chen D, Zhao CM. Tissue responses to hexyl 5-aminolevulinate-induced photodynamic treatment in syngeneic orthotopic rat bladder cancer model: possible pathways of action. J Biomed Opt. 2011;16(2):028001.

112. Ji HT, Chien LT, Lin YH, Chien HF, Chen CT. 5-ALA mediated photodynamic therapy induces autophagic cell death via AMP-activated protein kinase. Mol Cancer. 2010; 28;9:91.

113. Chaabane W, User SD, El-Gazzah M, Jaksik R, Sajjadi E, Rzeszowska-Wolny J, Los MJ. Autophagy, apoptosis, mitoptosis and necrosis: interdependence between those pathways and effects on cancer. Arch Immunol Ther Exp (Warsz). 2013;61(1):43-58.

114. Skulachev VP. Bioenergetic aspects of apoptosis, necrosis and mitoptosis. Apoptosis. 2006;11(4):473-85.

115. Vandenabeele P, Declercq W, Van Herreweghe F, Vanden Berghe T. The role of the kinases RIP1 and RIP3 in TNF-induced necrosis. Sci Signal. 2010 Mar 30;3(115):re4.

116. Degterev A, Huang Z, Boyce M, Li Y, Jagtap P, Mizushima N, Cuny GD, Mitchison TJ, Moskowitz MA, Yuan J. Chemical inhibitor of nonapoptotic cell death with therapeutic potential for ischemic brain injury. Nat Chem Biol. 2005 ;1(2):112-9.

117. Festjens N, Vanden Berghe T, Cornelis S, Vandenabeele P. RIP1, a kinase on the crossroads of a cell's decision to live or die. Cell Death Differ. 2007 Mar;14(3):400-10.

118. Chavez-Valdez R, Martin LJ, Northington FJ. Programmed Necrosis: A Prominent Mechanism of Cell Death following Neonatal Brain Injury. Neurol Res Int. 2012;2012:257563.

119. Wu W, Liu P, Li J. Necroptosis: an emerging form of programmed cell death.Crit Rev Oncol Hematol. 2012;82(3):249-58.

120. Coupienne I, Fettweis G, Piette J. RIP3 expression induces a death profile change in U2OS osteosarcoma cells after 5-ALA-PDT. Lasers Surg Med. 2011;43(7):557-64.

121. Coupienne I, Fettweis G, Rubio N, Agostinis P, Piette J. 5-ALA-PDT induces RIP3-dependent necrosis in glioblastoma. Photochem Photobiol Sci. 2011;10(12):1868-78.

122. Warnakulasuriya S. Causes of oral cancer--an appraisal of controversies. Br Dent J. 2009;2;207(10):471-475.

123. van der Waal I, Schepman KP, van der Meij EH. A modified classification and staging system for oral leukoplakia. Oral Oncol. 2000;36(3):264-6.

124. Lodi G, Porter S. Management of potentially malignant disorders: evidence and critique. J Oral Pathol Med. 2008;37(2):63-9.

125. Lodi G, Sardella A, Bez C, Demarosi F, Carrassi A. Interventions for treating oral leukoplakia. Cochrane Database Syst Rev. 2006 18;(4):CD001829.

126. Jerjes W, Hamdoon Z, Hopper C. Photodynamic therapy in the management of potentially malignant and malignant oral disorders. Head Neck Oncol. 2012 ;30;4:16.

127. Quon H, Grossman CE, Finlay JC, Zhu TC, Clemmens CS, Malloy KM, Busch TM.Photodynamic therapy in the management of pre-malignant head and neck mucosal dysplasia and microinvasive carcinoma. Photodiagnosis Photodyn Ther. 2011;8(2):75-85.

128. Chen HM, Chen CT, Yang H, Lee MI, Kuo MY, Kuo YS, Wang YP, Tsai T, Chiang CP. Successful treatment of an extensive verrucous carcinoma with topical 5-aminolevulinic acid-mediated photodynamic therapy. J Oral Pathol Med. 2005 ;34(4):253-256.

129. Chen HM, Yu CH, Tu PC, Yeh CY, Tsai T, Chiang CP. Successful treatment of oral verrucous hyperplasia and oral leukoplakia with topical 5-aminolevulinic acid-mediated photodynamic therapy. Lasers Surg Med. 2005;37(2):114-122.

130. Sieroń A, Adamek M, Kawczyk-Krupka A, Mazur S, Ilewicz L. Photodynamic therapy (PDT) using topically applied delta-aminolevulinic acid (ALA) for the treatment of oral leukoplakia. J Oral Pathol Med. 2003;32(6):330-336.

131. Chen HM, Chen CT, Yang H, Kuo MY, Kuo YS, Lan WH, Wang YP, Tsai T, Chiang CP. Successful treatment of oral verrucous hyperplasia with topical 5-aminolevulinic acid-mediated photodynamic therapy. Oral Oncol. 2004;40(6):630-637.

132. Lin HP, Chen HM, Yu CH, Yang H, Wang YP, Chiang CP. Topical photodynamic therapy is very effective for oral verrucous hyperplasia and oral erythroleukoplakia. J Oral Pathol Med. 2010;39(8):624-630.

133. J Jerjes W, Upile T, Hamdoon Z, Mosse CA, Akram S, Hopper C. Photodynamic therapy outcome for oral dysplasia. Lasers Surg Med. 2011;43(3):192-199.

134. Jerjes W, Upile T, Hamdoon Z, Alexander Mosse C, Morcos M, Hopper C. Photodynamic therapy outcome for T1/T2 N0 oral squamous cell carcinoma. Lasers Surg Med. 2011;43(6):463-469.

135. Barcessat AR, Huang I, Rabelo GD, Rosin FC, Ferreira LG, de Cerqueira Luz JG, Corrêa L. Systemic toxic effects during early phases of topical 4-NQO-induced oral carcinogenesis in rats. J Oral Pathol Med. 2014;43(10):770-777.

136. Schoop RA, Noteborn MH, Baatenburg de Jong RJ. A mouse model for oral squamous cell carcinoma. J Mol Histol. 2009;40(3):177-181

137. Srinivasan P, Sabitha KE, Shyamaladevi CS. Modulatory efficacy of green tea polyphenols on glycoconjugates and immunological markers in 4-Nitroquinoline 1-oxide-induced oral carcinogenesis-A therapeutic approach. Chem Biol Interact. 2006;25;162(2):149-156.

138. Sioga A, Economou L, Kaklamanos EG, Antoniades V, Keramidas G, Manthos A,Antoniades K. Ultrastructural changes of the palatal mucosa following application of 4-nitroquinoline-l-oxide (4NQO) in rats subjected to major salivary gland excision. Oral Surg Oral Med Oral Pathol Oral Radiol Endod. 2006;101(4):487-498.

139.. Emilio C.Comparison of the efficacy of aminolevulinic acid with that of its methyl ester using photodynamic therapy in the treatment of feline squamous cell carcinoma. [thesis] Sâo Paulo: Universidade de Sâo Paulo, Instituto de Pesquisas Energéticas e Nucleares, 2008

140. Mallia RJ, Subhash N, Sebastian P, Kumar R, Thomas SS, Mathews A,

Madhavan J. In vivo temporal evolution of ALA-induced normalized fluorescence at different anatomical locations of oral cavity: application to improve cancer diagnostic contrast and potential. Photodiagnosis Photodyn Ther. 2010 Sep;7(3):162-175.

141. Chen X, Zhao P, Chen F, Li L, Luo R. Effect and mechanism of 5-aminolevulinic acid-mediated photodynamic therapy in esophageal cancer. Lasers Med Sci. 2011;26(1):69-78

142. Schneider CA, Rasband WS, Eliceiri KW. NIH Image to ImageJ: 25 years of image analysis. Nat Methods. 2012 ;9(7):671-675.

143. Nakaseko H, Kobayashi M, Akita Y, Tamada Y, Matsumoto Y. Histological changes and involvement of apoptosis after photodynamic therapy for actinic keratoses. Br J Dermatol. 2003;148(1):122-127.

144. Yu CH, Chen HM, Hung HY, Cheng SJ, Tsai T, Chiang CP. Photodynamic therapy outcome for oral verrucous hyperplasia depends on the clinical appearance, size, color, epithelial dysplasia, and surface keratin thickness of the lesion. Oral Oncol. 2008;44(6):595-600.

145. Xie Y, Wei ZB, Zhang Z, Wen W, Huang GW. Effect of 5-ALA-PDT on VEGF and PCNA expression in human NPC-bearing nude mice. Oncol Rep. 2009;22(6):1365-1371.

146. Chen HM, Chen CT, Yang H, Lee MI, Kuo MY, Kuo YS, Wang YP, Tsai T, Chiang CP. Successful treatment of an extensive verrucous carcinoma with topical 5-aminolevulinic acid-mediated photodynamic therapy. J Oral Pathol Med. 2005;34(4):253-256.

147. Chen HM, Chen CT, Yang H, Kuo MY, Kuo YS, Lan WH, Wang YP, Tsai T, Chiang CP. Successful treatment of oral verrucous hyperplasia with topical 5-aminolevulinic acid-mediated photodynamic therapy. Oral Oncol.2004 ;40(6):630-637.

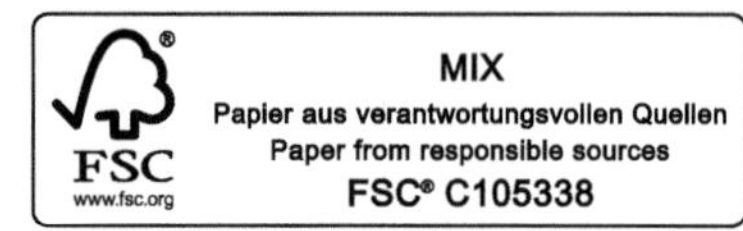

Printed by Books on Demand GmbH, Norderstedt / Germany